Robert

It's an honor to have
you as a friend.

HEADACHE

Finding the Underlying Cause

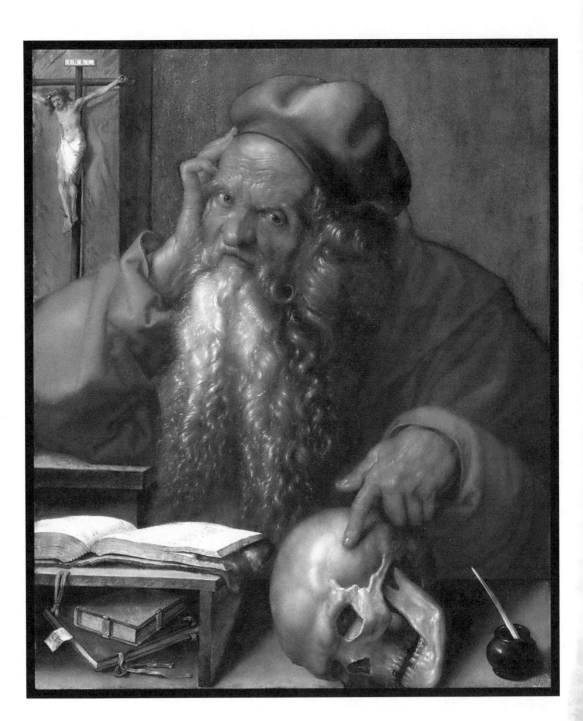

HEADACHE

Finding the Underlying Cause

David Nelson Smith, MD, PhD

NewCastle Press
Rochester, New York

St. Jerome by Albrecht Dürer 1521

Considered the greatest German artist of the Renaissance, Dürer was an innovator of many talents. Here St. Jerome is depicted in the last years of his life with one hand on his head and the other on a skull. Some say that he is pondering the brevity of life. At first glance, I saw an old man trying to understand his headaches, a fitting theme here. (Used with permission of the Portuguese Institute of Museums.)

Disclosure
The author has served as consultant and speaker for the major manufacturers of headache medications. Recognizing a possible conflict of interest, he no longer receives consulting fees, speaker fees, grants or other compensation from any drug manufacturer in any form. The writing, printing or promotion of this book has not received support from any pharmaceutical company.

ISBN 978-0-9887582-0-9

Library of Congress Control Number has been applied for.

NewCastle Press
Rochester, New York
www.newcastlepress.com
www.davidnelsonsmith.com

Printed in the USA
First Edition

Meet the Author

I began my career in 1960 when I was elected president of the American Junior Red Cross, a time when Red Cross was focused on leadership training. I went on to the Massachusetts Institute of Technology where I received a Bachelors of Science in electrical engineering, then New York University for a Masters of Science in electrical engineering. At that time my interests were electronic circuit design and statistical communications theory, the science of extracting signals from noise.

I went on to medical school at the University of Rochester Medical Center where I also began studies for a PhD in neuroanatomy. Biomedical engineering had yet to become a discipline. My dream was to apply engineering principles to core problems in medicine. The dream became reality when the Life Insurance Medical Research Fund awarded a full scholarship for my MD and PhD studies to do just this.

Medical school was followed by an internship in medicine, then residency in neurology at the University of Rochester Medical Center, where in 1977 I entered practice as an instructor in neurology and ophthalmology. I established the first evoked response laboratory in Rochester, designing the electronic equipment myself. Evoked responses extract sensory signals from the noise of EEG. They had become a key study in the diagnosis of multiple sclerosis. I received a PhD in anatomy and then went on to a postdoctoral fellowship in neuro-ophthalmology at Harvard's Massachusetts Eye and Ear Infirmary. I returned to the URMC as assistant professor to establish the medical center's neuro-ophthalmology service, and became board certified in neurology in 1986.

In 1989 I left the University for private practice where I had an opportunity for another postdoctoral fellowship, this time with Dr. George Engel, focused on the doctor-patient relationship using Engel's biopsychosocial approach to patient care.

Hardly a day goes by without a patient asking, "What ever made you go from engineering to medicine?" With a bit of humor I'll say, "I like to figure things out. Isn't that what engineers do?" It's just too painful to face the truth.

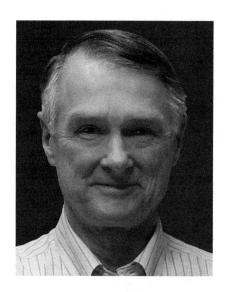

My brother Bobby was shot to death by a "friend" when he was 15 years old. Looking back over my life, I can see now that caring for those who are ill has been my way of trying to undo what happened in those few minutes in 1945. I'm trying to do the good in this world that Bobby would have done, had he lived. Only in recent years have I become aware of this.

I've been called a true renaissance man. Beyond the BS and MS in engineering, the MD and PhD, board certification in neurology and postdoctoral training in neuro-ophthalmology, I have keen interests in neuro-imaging, multiple sclerosis, electrodiagnostics, neuroimmunology, headache, and undiagnosed and rare diseases, all with an uncommon awareness of the human element. My life's focus has been patient care.

In *Headache: Finding the Underlying Cause* I contend that we suffer from headache because the diagnosis is usually flawed in some way and that our suffering need not be. Most headaches are easily diagnosed and easily treated. I show how it's done and go on to explain why some fail to improve and how we can turn those failures into success.

In the pages that follow you will see what might be called "an MIT approach to headache," written by a physician with 35 years of clinical experience. I hope you find this, my first book, to be of value.

David Nelson Smith, MD, PhD

Dedicated, with a deep sense of gratitude, to my patients who have brought so many challenging stories and have been a source of inspiration and wisdom beyond imagination.

Contents

List of Stories

About this Book

For clarity, I've organized this book as if it were a thesis: " Here's the question. Here's what I did. Here's what I found."

Chapter One asks the *Question*, Chapter Two states the *Method*, Chapters Three, Four and Five are the *Results*, Chapters Six, Seven and Eight are the *Discussion* and Chapter Nine is the *Conclusion* I draw from all of this.

However, I want to make it clear that this is not a formal research study. Although most of the stories are documented in the patients' charts, some of the most instructive stories took place years ago. I offer them from my best recall. Please understand that even a well-documented story is an *interpreted* kind of data. Different individuals see different things in the same story. So I cannot claim that what I'm about to say is rigorous in the sense of evidence-based medicine. Ultimately you must be the judge of its value.

How to use this book

The ideas build upon one another, so you will have the best understanding by reading from beginning to end. Key points are emphasized as callouts in the outside margin. Footnotes are located in the bottom outside margin in small print. You can quickly get an overview of the book in one sitting by first reading the Contents page. Then simply read the callouts as you page through the book. That offers an overview before the reading begins in earnest.

Who's the audience?

Nearly everyone who reviewed the manuscript asked this question. In engineering, this book would be called a *horizontal application*. Any software application that targets a large number of users with different knowledge and skill sets is called a horizontal application. The reviewers had a broad range of backgrounds, and they all seemed to get something out of it.

I hope you will not be offended by my use of the term "doctor" rather than "physician's assistant," "nurse practitioner," "health care provider" or any number of other terms applied to those who provide health care. What follows applies broadly, of course. It is not restricted to "doctors."

Disclaimer

This is not a self-help book. It is intended as education only, offered with the firm belief that a better understanding of headache will hasten anyone's return to health. Professional medical care was required in every case reported here. The author assumes no liability for the content in this book or its interpretation and application.

Acknowledgements

I am deeply indebted to many individuals who so graciously contributed to the production of this book. Above all, Thank you Kevin Billett for the cover design and book layout. Thank you Rachel Washburn for editing.

Thank you to Ellie, Josh, Jack, Beth, Elaine, Ed, Paul, Tony and to the reviewers for your thoughts and comments. You have my sincere appreciation.

Chapter One

A Pointed Question

A simple question begins an inquiry that yields some uncommon insight.

No matter how you look at it, most headaches are not serious, and most are easy to diagnose. On top of that, we have effective treatment today for nearly every kind of headache. Why then do so many of us continue to suffer with headache? Why is life so much less than it could be? Why are our dreams in life crippled by them and why must we continue to pay the high price, not only by the person who suffers, but also by spouse, employer, and our society as a whole?

Most headaches are not serious. They are easy to diagnose and have effective treatments. Why then do so many of us continue to suffer with headache?

When a person comes with headaches they've had for a long time, the story often begins: "I've seen so many doctors . . ." I'm encouraged to see that they are still trying to find an answer, but right up front, I let them know that my approach will be different from the others, and I need them to buy into the idea. It usually goes something like this:

> *Engineer:* "I hope you understand that I'm an engineer. What engineers do, they like to figure things out, take something apart and see how it works. I'm even glad, in a way, that you're having your headaches now. If you weren't having symptoms, my ability to figure this all out would be sorely limited. I don't want to focus on treatment, because we don't even know what we'd be treating. Everything I do until the last visit is for diagnosis. I don't focus on treatment because once we know, thoroughly and correctly, how the headaches come to be, then the treatment is obvious; or as they say at MIT, it's "intuitively obvious to the most casual observer." As far

as I'm concerned, treatment is just part of the diagnosis. Until we're certain of the diagnosis, even the medications that I prescribe are given for diagnostic purposes, not for treatment. I learn a great deal about what's causing your headaches from the way a person responds to various medications."

I'll be taking a degree in medicine and another in engineering, and putting them together to take a fresh look at headaches of all kinds.

So I'm asking you, dear reader, to buy into my approach as well. At least give it serious consideration. What we're going to be doing here is not like any headache book that you've ever read. I want to say this loud and clear. I'll be taking a degree in medicine and another in engineering, and putting them together to take a fresh look at headaches of all kinds so that we can understand them in a way that truly allows you to find well-being.

———

In the pages that follow, you will see how I found the answer to the opening question: "Why do so many of us continue to suffer with headaches?" If you've tried other approaches, and you still have headaches, read on.

Chapter Two

Learning from Success

A patient, whose headaches are not fazed by eliminating all food triggers, prompts me to examine the charts of patients who got better. I make a fascinating discovery: why the headaches defied a cure for so long in the first place.

As I see it, there are three kinds of headache. The most common, by far, are what we might call *benign headaches.* By this I mean that they do not have serious medical consequences or threaten life. I call them benign even though they are far from benign when we consider the amount of suffering and incapacitation they cause. Then there are *serious headaches*, which may have serious consequences, but fortunately are not common. Finally there are *baffling headaches*, which are more common than you might think. To begin, let's turn our attention to the most common headache known to man, migraine. Fortunately it's one of the benign headaches.

As we proceed, keep in mind the difference between the word *headache* and the word *migraine.* Headache refers to any kind of pain that happens in the head and neck. Migraine is one specific kind of headache.

As I see it, there are three kinds of headache: benign, serious and baffling. The most common headache known to man is migraine. Fortunately it is benign.

Barking up the Wrong Tree

Migraine is one of the benign headaches and is, by far, the most common kind of headache known to man. Traditionally, treatment begins by eliminating food triggers, although this may not be the answer for everyone.

Rice and Water: Some years ago, I saw a man in his forties for a troublesome pattern of headache. He was an intelligent fellow, an engineer as I recall. The headaches were migraine, no doubt about it, so I gave him a trigger list and suggested that he avoid these foods because they were generally thought to trigger migraine. At the time, I had the trigger list printed up as a tri-fold brochure because I handed it out so often.

Two or three weeks later he returned visibly upset. Trying to contain himself, through clenched teeth, he said, "Dr. Smith, I've had nothing to eat for three weeks but rice and water. Why am I still getting headaches?"

Cleverly, my patient had removed all possible food triggers in one fell swoop, just as one might do in search of a food allergy. He had proved beyond any question that red wine, fermented cheese, MSG, chocolate, and so on, were not the cause of *his* headaches. Something else was causing his headaches, something not on my trigger list.

> **Cleverly, my patient had removed all possible food triggers in one fell swoop. Something else was causing his headaches, something not on my trigger list.**

He never returned, so I never had a chance to figure out the cause of his headaches, but he did leave me with a tantalizing question: Was I barking up the wrong tree by trying to fix his headaches with my trigger list?

When the fellow asked "Why am I still getting headaches?" the truth was that I didn't know, although he was certainly asking the right question, the question "Why?" That word implies there is something deeper, something we still need to uncover. How could I find out what it was?

> **"I'll search through my patients' charts, those who had succeeded in getting rid of their headaches. What was it that made them better?"**

Then I got an idea. I'll search through my patients' charts, those who had succeeded in getting rid of their headaches. What was it that made them better? What had changed? That should give me some answers.

Two Sets of Three

So I tossed my trigger lists and began to look through the success stories. What I found was something much more important than my ineffective trigger lists.

Six factors, what I call *two sets-of-three*, popped up in case after case. They weren't triggers in the sense that one does something and then a headache quickly follows. The two sets-of-three are better thought of as activators because they are ongoing things that tend to make migraine more likely to happen. When the activators for a particular person were found and treated, the headaches improved dramatically. A few foods did prove to be potent activators, but most of the things on my trigger lists were only weak activators of migraine. They were not the answer for most people.

We found the greatest gain when we focused on the two sets-of-three. I think of the first set-of-three as *the first pass* and the second set as *the second pass.*

The first pass

The first set-of-three migraine activators are 1) alcohol in any form, 2) pushing through the day with caffeine and 3) using painkillers every day. I hate to say this now, but in those days I often said to my patient, "This first pass is under your control more than it is mine. So go fix these things. Stop the alcohol and the pain medications and quit pushing through the day with a pot of coffee. Come back if you're still getting headaches."

Now, I realize that a person uses alcohol and caffeine and pain killers for a reason. Take smoking for example. If I ask, "Why do you smoke? What does a smoke do for you?" One person might say, "It calms me." Another, "When I light up, I get a lift. It gets me going." I'm left wondering, "How are we ever going to get this person off tobacco if we don't first fix the nervous feeling inside that needs calming or the lack of get-up-and-go that needs a pick-me-up?" Now, even with the things in the first pass that I used to give back to the patient, I try to help as best I can. I know there are good reasons behind the drinking, the caffeine and taking pills for pain.

I've since simplified the first pass. Generally, anything that's habit-forming is suspect because addictive substances have withdrawal symptoms. A number of these bring on a rebound headache when they are discontinued.

For example, if you take an opiate like Vicodan or Percocet[1] every day, then after a few days the medication doesn't seem to help. You have to take more to get the same relief because the brain's opiate receptors quickly become less sensitive to opiates. The more you take the less sensitive your receptors become. Then if you stop the opiate, even for 12 hours or so, the pain suddenly becomes much worse than it was in the first place. The potent painkillers that you'd been taking have desensitized the opiate receptors in your brain. Therefore, your body's natural opiates now

> **For migraine, we had the greatest gain when we focused on the strong factors activating the headaches. Trying to eliminate weak factors only diverts our attention from where the focus needs to be.**

1. **Vicodan and Percodan** are combination medications in which hydrocodone or oxycodone are combined with aspirin or Tylenol. The codone component is a synthetic codeine-like narcotic that provides most of the pain relief.

have little effect. This is classic *analgesic rebound*. It's a common cause of perpetual headache.

In a similar way habit-forming sedatives cause agitation and sleep disturbance when they are withdrawn. Alcohol and the butalbital in Fiorinol have similar withdrawal symptoms. Caffeine, tobacco, anxiety medications, even marijuana, have their own withdrawal symptoms. Discontinuing any of them seems to disturb the body's equilibrium, which tends to make migraine more likely to occur in a person who is susceptible to migraine.

Second pass

The second set-of-three migraine activators are 1) depletion, 2) strong emotions and 3) female hormones. This is where I focus my efforts in the clinic. By depletion, I mean exhaustion. Strong emotions and changes in female hormones are obvious enough. We'll see how these three activators play out in the stories that follow, but the point I want to make here is that depletion, emotions, and female hormones express themselves in a style that's unique to the individual and the life in which that person is embedded. This means that there are as many different ways to activate migraine as there are people who have them. As you will see, there are common styles or patterns to the way migraine is activated that make it easier to identify the underlying cause.

Depletion, strong emotions and female hormones, this is where I focus my efforts.

It seems that whenever I mention female hormones, the next thing I hear is, "Oh, I'd really like to hear more about that." Just about every cell in the female body has estrogen receptors. Hormonal changes are not only responsible for puberty and menopause, they also cause PMS (premenstrual syndrome) which is a collection of physical symptoms, emotional changes and, you guessed it, headache. The headaches are usually migraine, and they're probably caused by the same thing that triggers the menses: a precipitous drop in estrogen and progesterone levels.

These hormones explain why migraine typically begins with puberty and ends with menopause. There's even a special name for migraine that occurs every month at the start of the menses: *catamenial migraine*. If your migraine began with puberty and occur every month with your menses, you can figure there's a strong hormonal component.

Here's the problem: One woman says, "I only get migraine when I'm pregnant." Another says, "The only time my migraine goes away is when I'm pregnant." It's the same with oral contraceptives;

they help migraine in some women, and make it worse in others. In my hands, attempts to treat catamenial migraine are, well let's say, unpredictable. To be perfectly honest, I find female hormones a bit intimidating.

It might help to use an oral contraceptive or discontinue the pill, if you're already on one. A low-dose estrogen patch can be applied just before the menses begin. This moderates the rapid drop in estrogen level that induces the menses and activates migraine. Some women find it helpful to use an extended-cycle oral contraceptive, so they only have menses three or four times a year.

As a rule, migraine moderates considerably after menopause, although hormonal fluctuations during the transition to menopause may worsen the headache pattern for a time. Medically or surgically induced menopause is less predictable. I generally do not recommend this as a treatment for migraine. Just because one of these hormonal manipulations works for one woman does not mean that it will help another.

I prefer to work on depletion and emotions first, hoping that we won't have to face the hormones. As these activators improve, a person becomes less susceptible to migraine in general. We might even hear something like "You know, when I sleep, I don't get those awful headaches every month."

Activators More Than Triggers

There is no question that many items on my trigger lists are potent migraine activators. Red wine and hard liquor, especially enough to get a little buzz, are infamous. It's not unusual to hear that a glass of red wine with dinner was followed by a knock-down migraine an hour or so later. More often though, alcohol in any form, even in modest amounts, does not immediately trigger a headache. Rather, it seems to destabilize the migraine process in the sense that trivial things make the headache happen more easily, more frequently and more severely, without a clear one-to-one correlation. Pushing through the day with caffeine and using an analgesic every day are behaviors that tend to make migraine unstable in a similar way. I like to think of such things as *activators*, rather than triggers. They make migraine more likely to happen.

It can be hard to see cause and effect when a glass of wine, for example, doesn't immediately trigger a migraine. Then we might

Many items on my trigger lists do not immediately trigger a headache. They destabilize the migraine process so that trivial things make migraine happen more easily without a clear one-to-one correlation. So I think of them as activators, rather than triggers.

easily dismiss wine as the prime suspect and miss the opportunity to make a helpful change. I see this, for example, when a person does not get restorative sleep. Even though poor sleep is a potent activator of migraine, many people are surprisingly unable to see the connection.

Without an immediate cause and effect, how do we find out what's activating the migraine? That's easy; we use a principle from statistical communication theory: the *cross-correlation function*. Here's how it works.

> *Connoisseur:* A well-to-do fellow with insufferable headaches was drinking two glasses of red wine every night with dinner. When I suggested that he do a "no alcohol for two weeks" experiment, an uneasy look came to his face.
>
> "I have a few hundred bottles in my wine cellar. I just can't do that. I'm a connoisseur."
>
> "Then try drinking three glasses with dinner every night and see if the headaches get worse."
>
> I never saw him after that. I think he knew the answer.

Here's another common way we can use cross-correlation. One of the first things I ask when a person comes for headaches is, "Do you sleep?" If they say, "Not well." Then what I need to know is, "If you sleep, do you get headaches?"

Even though poor sleep is a potent activator of migraine, many people are surprisingly unable to see the connection.

We can use the cross-correlation technique to answer this question. The patient might take a sleeping pill for two weeks. Does the pill give you a good night's rest? If so, when you get a good night's sleep, do you still get headaches? If you're still not sure, then go through another cycle or two, on the sleeping pill for two weeks, then off for two weeks. That should clear up any question.

Strong and Weak Factors

I agree with the *Rice and Water* fellow. Avoiding food triggers doesn't get many people very far with their migraine. I don't mean to say that chocolate, MSG, tyramine and aspartame, to name a few, do not trigger or activate migraine. They do in many people, but we are not likely to feel well simply by avoiding what are commonly called triggers; most of the time they have only a weak effect in activating our migraine.

Trying to eliminate these *weak factors* only diverts our attention from where the focus needs to be: on the *strong factors*. Almost always there are other things activating the migraine, things less obvious, but much more important. By strong factors I mean specific ways that an individual experiences depletion, emotions and hormones. When we identify and correct the strong factors, the headaches are more likely to improve, and the sensitivity to food triggers, light, and smells improves as well. Identifying the strong factors activating migraine is the key to feeling truly well.

Here's another way to say this: When foods and allergies and fluorescent lights and the weather seem to trigger your migraine, when you are perpetually sensitive to light or have chronic eyestrain, it simply means one thing: you are a migraine trying to happen. In other words, you are lingering at migraine threshold all the time. A person will say right out, "Every little thing gives me a headache." If I wear a striped shirt in the office that day, if I even look at them cross-eyed, it's "Oh, you're giving me a headache!"

> **When every little thing gives you a migraine, it means you are lingering at migraine threshold. You're a migraine trying to happen.**

Be forewarned, however. A person's strong factors may not be easy to change, which is one reason some individuals just never seem to get better. However, when a person succeeds in improving the important activators, even by a little, they might find that they can have some alcohol, or even have their menses, without a headache. If you are trying to control your headaches by living in incandescent lighting or following a meticulous diet, you are probably working on weak factors. Chances are you're wasting your time. When you find the strong factors and fix them, you won't have a problem with bright light or your menses or Christmas shopping; and you'll probably be able to have champagne on New Year's Eve, in moderation of course.

> **If you do not inherit a susceptibility to migraine, then you can drink alcohol all you want, have terrible sleep, you can have off-the-wall emotions, and you won't get a headache.**

Susceptible, but Headache Free

One last thing about migraine activators: If you do not inherit a susceptibility to migraine, then you can drink alcohol all you want, have terrible sleep . . . you can have off-the-wall emotions, and you won't get a headache. You may have other problems, but not migraine. I've had migraine since I was ten years old. I'm highly susceptible. My father was not. I can remember him saying, "I don't know what a headache is. I've never had one."

A corollary to the "you must be susceptible to get migraine" principle is this: Even though you are susceptible, if you find and

> **Even though a person is susceptible, if you find and correct the activators, the strong factors, you can be virtually headache-free.**

correct the activators, the strong factors that is, you can be virtually headache-free. The challenge is finding them.

I've been essentially headache-free for years now, because I get good sleep. All I need is something to keep me from sleeping and I'm right back into my old migraine pattern.

The Answer is in the Story

Why did I turn to the stories of my patients? Why not read a book by an expert? Scour the journals? How about doing a study myself, just to prove beyond any shadow of doubt how effective or ineffective treatment-by-trigger-list really is? I didn't need a controlled study to prove that trigger lists don't work. I was already sure of that.

> *Only 20 Minutes:* A few months after I started neurology residency, I was in the emergency department at the end of the day, swamped with patients, two to be exact. One of them was a patient of Dr. Joynt's, the chair of the department and a very wise clinician.
>
> Dr. Joynt came down to see his patient before he left for the day. As I presented the case, he quickly sensed the tension in my voice. In his fatherly way, he looked me straight in the eye over the top of his glasses, and with a little smile said, "David, if you only have twenty minutes to see a patient, spend nineteen minutes on the history, one minute on the exam, and no minutes on the EEG." (This was in 1974. It would be a few years before we had our first CT scanner.)

In his gentle way, Dr. Joynt was trying to say that we find the answers in the story more often than in the exam or tests. Now, 35 years later, this still holds true. Even with the latest MRI technology, I find that the answers still come mostly from the patient's history.

Dr. Joynt was trying to say that we find the answers in the story more often than in the exam or tests.

That's why I turned to the patient records when I lost faith in my trigger lists. I wanted to learn something new, so I went straight to the source: the patient's experience.

In those stories I found a gold mine of information. During 35 years of practice, I've seen many thousands of patients, so I had many stories in this resource. Mostly the patients I see are loaded on the refractory end of the spectrum. I don't see many ordinary cases. More often they're individuals who aren't getting better.

They're dilemmas in some way. Another name for diagnostic medicine is *the buck stops here.*

I was curious about those who in fact *did* get better. What finally fixed the headache? I began to see patterns, the two sets-of-three, for example. To my surprise, I found something I wasn't even looking for, something far more important than the cure. I found what it was that prevented them from finding the answer in the first place. I found what kept them ill, often for years.

Out of this came a whole new way of thinking about headache, a new way to treat headache, and especially a new way of talking to my patients about their headaches. I used stories in a way that helped them see just how it is that they get headache. The very stories that taught me so much, I passed along to my patients as a poignant way of giving memorable counsel.

Now as I talk to a patient, I find myself telling them about what I've seen; how others like them found the answers and became well, and above all, I tell them about the lessons I've learned. Many times I've said to a discouraged patient, "If you could have hovered above my office for the past 35 years, you would have seen many ways that others have come to understand and fix what you may think is an impossible problem." The stories, call them case studies if you wish, provide a kind of credibility. After all, case reports are a form of scientific data.

I wanted to learn something new, so I went straight to the source: the patient's experience.

Even so, I don't tell these stories to my patients because they represent a form of evidence-based medicine. I tell them as stories because they are remarkably informative, interesting, understandable, memorable and enjoyable, and especially because they are so strongly personal and rich with insight. I often hear a patient comment, "You're talking about me there, Dr. Smith." A person can identify with a story and can better understand themselves through the experience of others.

These stories have also been an uncommon gift of learning for me. I would even venture to say that what I've learned from those for whom I've cared has been more important to diagnosis and treatment than what I've learned from the books and journals. Just look at the fellow with the rice and water diet. His clever approach not only showed me the shortcomings of the triggers concept, it sent me to work trying to understand things of much more substance: what finally brought them to an end, and why the headaches defied diagnosis and treatment for so long in the first place, often years. Using stories like this to convey an idea is a form of speaking in metaphor. It has become a powerful way to convey an idea in a simple and easily understood manner.

In these success stories, I found answers to the question, "Why do so many of us continue to suffer with headaches?"

————

I want to share what I've learned with you. It's your key to getting better. The stories in the chapters that follow are not rare or even infrequent or unusual. I hear variations of them every day. You might even see yourself in one of them.

Chapter Three

Benign Headaches

Looking into six common headache stories, we begin to realize there's more to these headaches than meets the eye.

Let's see what we can learn from a few of the more common headache stories. Although not serious for the most part, they are beyond *consuming* in terms of time in the doctor's office, dollars, and misery.

Sinus Headaches and Masquerade Migraine

In referring a patient, one primary care physician went on to say, "Headaches are the bane of our existence." One of the most common headaches seen by PCP's and specialists alike is what they call "sinus headaches." The visit often goes something like this:

> *Sinus Headaches:* "Doc, I've had sinus headaches all my life. They run in my family. My mother gets them, and so do her brother and sister. I know they're sinus headaches because the pain is right over my sinuses and I get this green stuff running down the back of my throat. I call my doctor and tell him 'I've got another sinus infection,' he gives me an antibiotic and a decongestant, and they're gone in a day or two."
>
> "Why are you here then? I'm a neurologist, not a sinus doctor."
>
> "Well, I have sinus headaches all the time. I can't get off antibiotics, and they're just getting worse. Last month I had one so bad; I couldn't even go to work. I was home in bed all day. It even made me sick to my stomach. So my doctor sends me to an ear-nose-throat doctor. He did a

scan and tells me that my sinuses are clean as a whistle!"

Diagnosis by assumption

This fellow and many like him have migraine, not sinus headaches. An incapacitating headache that makes a person sick to his stomach and sends him to bed is far more likely to be migraine than sinus disease. Migraine is often felt as discomfort over the sinuses and naturally goes away in a day or two. What about the green stuff? Many people who don't have sinus disease complain of that. It probably comes from the nasal airway, not the sinuses. It wasn't the antibiotic that took the headache away. It went away on its own.

When this fellow finally realized that he had migraine, the end was in sight. All we had to do was find the activator, fix that, and his headaches were a thing of the past. Why was that so hard?

Just think for a minute. How far can a person get by trying to treat migraine with an antibiotic and a decongestant? The reason he didn't get better is that he was treating the wrong thing. He made an assumption, sinus disease, and his assumption was just plain wrong.

There's a lesson to be learned here: Diagnosis by assumption is often misdiagnosis. One problem with a wrong diagnosis is that it stops the search for the correct one. A diagnosis is a conclusion, an answer. If it's wrong, not only does it lead to the wrong treatment, it also obstructs progress toward the correct answer. Wouldn't it be better to say, "I have these headaches or eyestrain or whatever the symptom is. I'd sure like to know the cause" That would keep the investigation going until we finally find what it is that makes us well.

Most of the headaches that we call sinus headaches are not caused by sinus disease. Headaches over the sinuses usually prove to be migraine; but don't you wonder why it seems so easy to mistake migraine for something else?

Masquerade migraine

There are many variations of this phenomenon in which migraine is thought to be something else. I think of these variations as *masquerade migraine*.

A family of disorders: Migraine takes different forms because it isn't a single disorder. In the first paragraph of his

An incapacitating headache that makes a person sick to his stomach and sends him to bed is far more likely to be migraine than sinus disease

How far can a person get by trying to treat migraine with an antibiotic and a decongestant?

Diagnosis by assumption is often misdiagnosis. One problem with a wrong diagnosis is that it stops the search for the correct one.

book *On megrim, sick-headache and some allied disorders: A Contribution to the Pathology of Nerve-storms*[2], esteemed London physician Edward Liveing called migraine "a family of disorders." This insight came from clinical experience alone, caring for his patients.

Liveing published his book in 1873. Today we know of several neurological mechanisms linked together in this process we call migraine. They may occur singly or in any combination. They include a mechanism for the pain of migraine called the *trigeminovascular reflex*, a mechanism for sensitivity to light and sound and smell called *central sensitization* and a mechanism for slow auras called *spreading depression of Leão*. Less appreciated members of the migraine family of disorders are *vasospasm*, which creates brief, fast-onset, stroke-like symptoms, and an *autonomic mechanism* that creates nausea and vomiting and the ashen face of migraine. The migraine process may even occur with little or no headache, an entity so common that it's been given a special name: *migraine equivalent*.

How and why these neural mechanisms are tied together is not clear, but it is clear that migraine can take many forms other than a sick headache with nausea that makes us pull the drapes and go to bed. The form it takes depends on which neurological mechanisms are active in a particular person on a particular day. It's a challenge indeed, when a person has migraine symptoms with no headache, but this does occur, and it occurs often.

Eyestrain: By far, most of those who complain of eyestrain have migraine as the underlying cause. The twelve-year-old who comes in wearing bifocals for eyestrain, almost always has the eyestrain of migraine. Usually it's a young person who worries. As we will see, worry is a potent migraine activator in young people.

One clue that the eyestrain is really a form of migraine is that it's accompanied by excessive sensitivity to light. A person often begins their complaint of eyestrain by saying they can't read for more than 15 minutes because it bothers their eyes so much. Then, as they continue their story, one hand goes over their brow to shade their eyes from the overhead fluorescent lights. They sit there squinting because everything seems so bright.

During central sensitization the volume control is turned up on all sensations. I remember this well from my own migraine days. I would go to the movies, close my eyes and just listen because

2. Liveing E. *On megrim, sick-headache and some allied disorders: A Contribution to the Pathology of Nerve-storms. J and A Churchill London 1873. A reprint is available in the Classics of Neurology & Neurosurgery Library series, 1986, Gryphon Editions, Ltd, Birmingham, Alabama.*

watching the movie bothered my eyes so much.

Central sensitization even includes excessive sensitivity to touch. In my migraine days, just the touch of the sheets was so unpleasant that it made me kind of twitchy. I can understand when someone says "My headaches get so bad that even my hair hurts."

In my own experience, migraine usually proves to be the cause of "my normal headaches," allergy headaches, and a multitude of other symptoms including some strange ones like chronic dizziness. Look for associated symptoms that suggest migraine: eyestrain, sensitivity to light, sound, or smell, and nausea. They're a tip-off that migraine is the cause.

Fibromyalgia and restorative sleep

I wouldn't call fibromyalgia a form of masquerade migraine, although both fibromyalgia and migraine have much in common.

Fibromyalgia is a controversial and poorly understood disorder. One of my patients said, "It's something the doctor tells you when he doesn't know what's wrong." We had a good laugh. Then I told her about my theory of fibromyalgia and how her symptoms of fibromyalgia might help us find the cause of her headaches.

Only a symptom: Fibromyalgia, as we understand it today, is what we call a clinical diagnosis. It's a diagnosis made from a cluster of symptoms and a pattern of tender spots on the body. There's no lab test to verify the diagnosis.

Fibromyalgia is not a diagnosis in the true sense of the word. Knowing through and through means that we know the mechanism of the disease, its underlying cause, what's called pathogenesis.

The word diagnosis (dia + gnosis) literally means knowing through and through, so fibromyalgia is not a diagnosis in the true sense of the word. Knowing through and through, to me, means that we know the mechanism of the disease, its underlying cause, what's called *pathogenesis*. Fibromyalgia has a pathogenesis. The problem is, nobody knows what it is. So there's more than an element of truth in my patient's funny comment. Pathogenesis is an important concept because it keeps us focused on the underlying cause, which is where our attention needs to be.

The pain of fibromyalgia is longstanding and generalized, which means that it involves the upper and lower as well as the left and right sides of the body. There are 18 typical tender areas or trigger points, although it's more common in my experience for a person to say, "Everything hurts." If a person has pain in 11 or more trigger points, fibromyalgia warrants consideration.

Like migraine, fibromyalgia is more than just pain. I hear the same complaints in both disorders. "I just don't feel well." . . . "I'm tired all the time. I don't sleep well." . . . "I can't think clearly or remember things. It's like there's a fog in my brain."

Here's another similarity: We speak of migraine and fibromyalgia as if they were diagnoses, although it would be more helpful to think of them as symptoms that have many possible underlying causes. Isn't that interesting? They seem to have so much in common. Could they also have a common pathogenesis?

The symptoms of some disorders are so specific that a diagnosis can be made with reasonable certainty from the symptoms alone. Stroke, Parkinson's disease, and multiple sclerosis often have diagnostic symptoms like this. Not so with the symptoms of fibromyalgia. They are non-specific; they can be caused by any number of disorders. In other words, there is nothing about the symptoms that say, "This is fibromyalgia, not something else." Furthermore, if it's fibromyalgia, all the tests, bloodwork and CT/MRI scans are normal.

A chronic pain-state might cause migraine in one person and fibromyalgia in another.

A few years ago, all too often, I'd hear, "My rheumatologist said that I had seventeen of the eighteen tender points of fibromyalgia. 'It's a classic case. There's no treatment, so you'll just have to learn to live with it.'"

Now we have FDA-approved medications for fibromyalgia. In my hands, none of them have been what you'd call highly effective. That's because they treat the symptoms, not the cause. So, for the most part, I think that many of those with fibromyalgia are still learning to live with it.

A chronic state of pain: There are many reasons a person might have pain every day. We've already seen that one way to guarantee pain is to take pain-killers daily, which creates the pain-state called *analgesic rebound*.

In most cases of migraine or fibromyalgia, analgesic rebound is not the problem. Something else is causing the pain. Both migraine and fibromyalgia are pain disorders. Both are often associated with sleep problems - fascinating. Could they simply be two expressions of the same thing: a chronic state of pain? This leads to another question: Could it be that lack of restorative sleep somehow creates a chronic pain-state that activates both migraine and the symptoms of fibromyalgia?

Fibromyalgia has one telling characteristic. If a person has both fibromyalgia and migraine, when I fix the migraine, the fibromyalgia usually gets better. Migraine and fibromyalgia are common disorders, so they frequently occur together. If fixing the migraine cures the fibromyalgia, then whatever caused the migraine might also have activated fibromyalgia.

I propose a theory to explain how a chronic pain-state might cause migraine in one person and fibromyalgia in another: The two disorders may simply represent inherited differences in the way that a person experiences pain. One person is susceptible to pain in the head while another person has susceptibility to pain in the body. In other words, some individuals have inherited genes making them susceptible to migraine when their pain mechanisms aren't working properly. Others have genes that make them feel pain in their body, not their head, when their pain mechanisms aren't working. Still others have an inherited susceptibility to both pain in their head and pain in their body. So they have both migraine and fibromyalgia when their pain mechanisms don't function properly.

Restorative sleep: I focus on sleep because, in some mysterious way, exhaustion seems to make a person more susceptible to pain. For example, when a person has post-herpetic neuralgia, a form of nerve pain following shingles, the pain usually becomes worse toward the end of the day as the person gets tired. Anyone seems to be more resistant to pain of any kind after a good night's rest. I would even go as far as to say that correcting a sleep disorder is one of the most helpful things a person can do for pain of any kind. The medical literature supports this. The perpetual lack of restorative sleep seems to make anyone more susceptible to pain.

> **Correcting a sleep disorder is one of the most helpful things a person can do for pain of any kind.**

How could it be that sleep influences pain? Theories proposed by Jouvet and Stern and Morgane in the early '70s suggest that the various stages of sleep restore the chemistry of the brain. That chemistry includes the neurotransmitters that regulate mood, mediate pain, and allow us to think clearly and remember things. After a long day, I am physically, mentally, and emotionally exhausted. I'm less creative and I find it more difficult to solve a problem. Then after a sound, restorative night's sleep, which I always seem to get - one of my blessings in life - the next morning my brain is functioning with remarkable clarity.

On the other hand, when a person wakes in the morning and is not restored by a good night's sleep, it's like waking up with half a tank of gas in the brain. This deficiency in brain chemistry seems to cause more than just fatigue. It makes a person quarrelsome, forgetful, confused and prone to mistakes. I hear comments like, "I must have Alzheimer's disease. I can't remember a thing." . . . "There's a fog in my brain." . . . "I can't think or focus my attention. Do I have ADHD?" A person might even wake in a sour mood, what's called dysphoria, a mild form of depression. Not only that, any pain we have, for any reason, is amplified. Sounds a little like fibromyalgia, doesn't it?

We have so many medications to speed up and stimulate the brain, so many ways to improve focus of attention, but nothing beats a good nights sleep.

New treatment possibilities: Now listen to this: If migraine and fibromyalgia are two forms of the same thing, a chronic pain state, then a whole new world of treatment possibilities opens up. If they both have the same underlying cause, then it follows that a treatment that is highly effective for migraine should also prove highly effective for fibromyalgia. Now we would be treating the cause, not just symptoms.

Here's a word of caution. If you look to migraine treatments in the hope of curing your fibromyalgia, be careful. Aside from a chronic pain-state caused by lack of restorative sleep, there are many other ways that migraine can be activated. The same probably holds true for fibromyalgia. If we want a cure for fibromyalgia, then we must diligently search for the underlying cause, not just treat symptoms.

Who knows, maybe we don't have to "learn to live with it" after all.

Tension-Type Headache

Another benign headache adding to the bane of the primary care physician's existence is the tension-type headache. Considered to be muscular in origin, it goes by a number of different names. Tension headache and muscle contraction headache are the most common.

> **The puzzling thing about tension headaches is that they are hard to separate from migraine.**

The puzzling thing about tension headaches is that they are hard to separate from migraine. In pure form migraine is characterized by an often severe one-sided headache that occurs in attacks lasting a day or so, which then clears completely.

Associated symptoms often include nausea, and vomiting, and excessive sensitivity to light, sound, and smell. Auras of visual or other neurological symptoms sometimes occur.

Tension-type headache, on the other hand, is a less severe, chronic headache that feels like a tight band around the head without the associated symptoms of migraine.

Surveys show that tension-type headache is more common than migraine by far. In my practice, however, the most common headaches have features of both migraine and tension-type headache, what are called *mixed-pattern headaches*.

A personal experience

It isn't uncommon for a patient to ask, "Can migraine give you a headache every day?" Some years ago, at a meeting of the International Headache Society, I heard a renowned expert try to simplify the distinction between migraine and tension-type headache by saying, "If it's a headache every day, it isn't migraine." Today, the IHS has a new category of headache. It's called chronic daily migraine. So much for definitions.

Can migraine give you a headache every day? My own experience is a good example.

My own experience with headache is a good example.

My Story: I've had headaches since I was 10 years old. At that time, I only had them in the summer. Typically, we'd come home from a day at the beach at Seaside Heights. I would be upstairs, a little sun burnt, with a splitting headache, vomiting into the toilet, while everybody else was down in the kitchen having hot dogs and potato salad.

I grew up in Trenton, New Jersey where the summer temperature got well up into the 90s and the sun was intense, at least for me. All winter I was fine, no headache. It was heat and the sun that gave me migraine when I was young.

In my senior year of high school the migraine occurred every few weeks and I began to have a lingering headache in the back of my neck. There I was trying to get high grades in school so I could get into a good college *and* working 35 hours a week fixing TVs in a repair shop *and* I had to write a speech for the Red Cross Convention. To top that off, my English paper was due. I hadn't even started it. I walked around that year with a sick feeling in the pit of my stomach most of the time.

At MIT, in my early 20s, the migraine always occurred on Friday night. A group of Swedish young people had "adopted" me. We started the evening with a progressive dinner, going from house to house, stuffing ourselves with Swedish meatballs and lutfisk. As the evening went on, I could feel a headache growing in the back of my neck along the left trapezius. By the time I got back to the dorm, it had become a bad migraine centered in my left eye. Then I'd lose all that fine Swedish cooking.

It was the socializing more than the overeating. It's always been stressful for me to socialize, even with the Swedes, some of the best friends I ever had. The worst headaches were yet to come.

During my three years of neurology training, the headaches never went away. You cannot know how much I love the study of the brain, but training to be a neurologist was stressful. I seldom slept. For three years I had a continuous headache in my neck muscles. I was so sensitive to light that I wore two pair of sunglasses to drive. As I mentioned before, in a movie theater I'd close my eyes and just listen. The eyestrain was that bad.

Every week or so all this would quickly escalate into a typical migraine, again in my left eye. I remember having one of them when I was on-call in the hospital. The neck pain and headache and nausea and eyestrain had been increasing all that day. At two in the morning, I was admitting a patient from the emergency department, when suddenly I felt very sick. I took the patient's history, then said, "I'll be back in a few minutes." went to the on-call room, vomited, took a headache pill and laid down for a few minutes. Then I went back to finish up.

During those years in training, I thought I would never get rid of the eyestrain and the headache every day. After residency though, life was easy. I slept. It took a year or more for the continuous muscular headache, the eyestrain, the sensitivity to light and the migraine to go away. Gradually, though, this panoply of symptoms all abated. Now, at 70, I haven't had anything like this in years. Maybe it's age, but two other things have changed: I'm not easily stressed now, and I sleep like a baby.

You can see how the pattern of these benign headaches can change through a lifetime. A pattern like this is so common that it's been given a name: *transformed migraine*. This pattern starts out as episodic migraine, then gradually, over years, transforms into a chronic daily headache as the migraine characteristics drop away. In the transition, migraine are mixed with a muscular kind of pain, a pattern called mixed-pattern headaches.

A theory of mixed-pattern headache

I have a theory that explains why migraine and tension-type headaches so often occur together. It comes out of my own experience with headaches.

> *Curious Symptom:* I had a curious symptom during those bad three years of headache. It was a kind of noise I heard in my eyes, both eyes, most of the time.
>
> If you want to know what it sounds like, do a little experiment. When it's quiet at night and you lie in bed, before you go to sleep turn onto one side so your ear is pressed into the pillow. Slide the opposite hand under the pillow.
>
> Now clench your teeth or tighten the muscles of your hand under the pillow. You should hear the noise. When you relax your jaw or hand, the noise goes away. What you hear is the noise caused by the contraction of individual motor units.
>
> The contraction of any muscle is caused by electrical pulses sent out from motor neurons in the spinal cord. Each neuron connects to hundreds of muscle fibers. Large muscles are powered by hundreds of thousands of such motor units. The more motor units that fire, and the more frequently the pulses occur, the stronger the muscle contraction. This is called *recruitment*.
>
> The noise you hear with your ear on the pillow is the summation of many motor units contracting in your jaw or hand. I heard this same noise, but in my eyes, when I had those three years of mixed pattern headaches. I presume it came from the facial muscles around the eyes or the muscles that move the eyes. The question is, "How could this happen?"

We know that the pain of migraine is caused in part by

Inflammatory substances released during migraine also cause inflammation in the muscles of the head and neck.

inflammatory substances released from nerve endings. According to my theory of mixed-pattern headache, the inflammatory substances released during migraine also cause inflammation in the muscles of the head and neck. Then pain fibers in the muscle carry this signal to the spinal cord where it causes motor neurons to fire, which in turn creates sustained muscle contraction. This may explain how migraine, an inflammatory process, causes the tight painful muscles of tension-type headache.

This theory does not say that pure muscle contraction headaches do not exist. Sustained contraction of any muscle is painful. In pure muscle contraction headaches, the cause of the sustained contraction is most likely the tension we feel in our muscles when we are stressed. So the name *tension-type headache* makes sense to me

At one time I thought I could tell the difference between migraine and tension-type headache perfectly well, but I don't feel that way any more. I guess it's no surprise that my approach to headache has changed through the years.

Why the fuss?

Traditionally there have been treatments for migraine and different treatments for tension-type headache. If they are two different things, then that makes sense. What if they're not? Suppose they have a common origin?

If the most important part of treatment is knowing the underlying cause, then it doesn't matter whether it's migraine or tension-type headache or a mix of the two. What matters is the underlying cause. That's what we need to know, and that's what I need to treat.

So now I stay focused on finding the cause. I treat neither the migraine or the tension-type headache. I treat the cause. When the migraine improves, the muscular component usually improves as well.

Eventually, I think we'll find that the pathogenesis of migraine and tension-type headache are tied together in some fundamental way. If so, both might respond to the same treatment.

Eventually, I think we'll find that the pathogenesis of migraine and that of the associated tension-type headache are tied together in some fundamental way. If so, both might respond to the same treatment.

Basilar Artery Migraine

Returning to migraine that masquerades as something else,

the next story is about a form of migraine that's often incorrectly diagnosed.

When a person suddenly falls to the ground unconscious, the first thing that comes to mind is syncope, a drop in blood pressure for some reason. If an epileptic seizure was the cause, there would usually be shaking and an increase in muscle tone. Here's another cause of sudden loss of consciousness.

> *Real Go-getter:* Fifteen years ago, I saw a thirty-year-old woman from a small town two hours away. She was having episodes of sudden loss of consciousness, as often as once a week. The episodes might last a minute. There was no warning and no shaking to suggest a seizure. During one episode, someone took her pulse. It was strong, and her heart rate was normal, so she wasn't having syncope. She said that she just fell to the ground and had no recall of what happened during the minute that she was out.
>
> Then she added two important things: At other times her vision suddenly tunneled down in both eyes or went completely dark for about 20 seconds. At times, she had a headache shortly before or after these episodes.

Tunnel vision and headache associated with loss of consciousness or other brief stroke-like symptoms are markers for a form of migraine first reported by Bickerstaff in 1961. He was a pediatrician who described several children with sudden episodes of brainstem symptoms. He called the entity *basilar artery migraine.*[3]

Bickerstaff presumed that basilar artery migraine was caused by vasospasm in the posterior circulation of the brain, also known as the vertebrobasilar system. The vertebrobasilar system supplies blood to the brainstem, cerebellum, and the occipital lobes. They are areas that process eye movements, coordination, balance and vision. The brainstem also regulates consciousness, heart rate, blood pressure and respiration. Motor and sensory pathways pass through the brainstem on their way to and from the spinal cord. Many different kinds of neurological symptoms can occur when the vertebrobasilar system does not work properly. These include loss of consciousness, loss of vision, tunnel vision, double vision, severe vertigo, as well as weakness and sensory changes in the face, arms, and legs. All of these symptoms occur with the tempo of vasospasm: rapid onset within seconds and short duration, often

With or without headache, the loss of consciousness, tunnel vision or other brief stroke-like symptoms are markers for basilar artery migraine.

3. Bickerstaff ER. Basilar artery migraine. *Lancet.* 1961;1:15.

less than thirty seconds, seldom more than five minutes. Although in some cases, residual symptoms persist for days. They usually improve, but may never resolve completely, leaving a person wondering if they indeed had a small stroke. I've never seen signs of a stroke on the MRI scan with basilar artery migraine, even when the symptoms persist like this.

I ordered an EEG and MRI scan and started verapamil, a calcium channel blocker, to prevent vasospasm. She returned about ten days later to review the studies. No further episodes. As long as she stayed on verapamil, she didn't have episodes, but miss a few doses, and they came right back. This dramatic response to a calcium channel blocker is virtually diagnostic for the vasospasm of basilar migraine.

During the next few years, she would pop into the office now and then to say that she was doing well. She would always ask, "Why can't I get off verapamil? How long does this go on?"

Now here's the interesting part:

> A few years after I first saw her, she came back with a new question. She had left her pressure-cooker job as an advertising executive in northern New Jersey and moved back home to a quiet country town. "I ran out of verapamil and guess what? No headaches and no passing out or anything else. How come?"
>
> "Maybe you're under too much pressure in New Jersey." I suggested.

The last time I saw her, she was back in New Jersey in another pressure-cooker job, and the headaches and episodes had all come back. At last report, she was back on verapamil and "All's well." Stress is a powerful activator of basilar migraine. Remove the stress and the symptoms might just disappear.

The spectrum of a disorder

Basilar migraine is not uncommon. It often goes undiagnosed or misdiagnosed for years while the patient continues to have stroke-like attacks of brainstem symptoms and visual change. Often the loss of consciousness is misdiagnosed as epilepsy. The tip-off is that seizure medications don't help. A dramatic response to verapamil suggests vasospasm as the cause. Almost always, the symptoms of basilar artery migraine go away completely when the dose is right.

Basilar migraine is a little more complicated than just vasospasm in the basilar artery. The nature of the brainstem symptoms suggests that only small branches of the basilar artery go into spasm. When tunnel vision occurs without brainstem symptoms, larger vessels, the posterior cerebral arteries, could be in spasm. They supply blood to the occipital lobes where vision is processed. In most people, these vessels come off the top of the basilar artery.

Although the sudden onset of tunnel vision or complete loss of vision in both eyes are definite markers for basilar migraine, and they respond to verapamil, I cannot explain how they are caused by vasospasm. The visual symptoms usually occur alone, without brainstem symptoms. For this to happen there would have to be simultaneous vasospasm of *both* posterior cerebral arteries or the arteries in the vicinity of the optic chiasm, unlikely events.

There's a common sequence to the pathogenesis of basilar migraine. It begins with strong emotions, anxiety or anger, what we call the fight or flight response. This brings on a strong adrenaline response which, in turn, initiates the vasospasm. This sequence of events can be blocked at three points. Tranquilizers can be used to turn down the volume control on emotions. Beta blockers decrease the adrenaline effect. Finally, calcium channel blockers, verapamil for example, block the vasospasm directly.

Without an appreciation for the spectrum of a disorder, it may be a long time before someone finally catches on.

Basilar artery migraine is part of the spectrum of migraine phenomena. Without an appreciation for the spectrum of a disorder, it can be a long time, filled with plenty of grief, before someone finally catches on. *Go-getter* was a quick fix because I had seen many variants of basilar migraine. When we appreciate the many forms that a disorder can take, and especially if we've been around long enough to have actually seen many of them, then the diagnosis can be made with a snap of the fingers.

Blood vessels in the posterior circulation of the brain, the vertebrobasilar system, are remarkably sensitive to vasospasm in a way that the anterior circulation, the carotid system, is not. As a rule, vasospasm causes brainstem and occipital symptoms, not carotid symptoms.

There's one exception. The blood vessels of the retina, supplied by the carotids, are exquisitely sensitive to vasospasm. When retinal artery vasospasm occurs, a person has partial or complete loss of vision in one eye with the fast vascular tempo as basilar artery migraine. This is often called *retinal migraine,* to make it clear that this is not the more common slowly evolving visual aura of migraine. This common visual aura is caused by a process called *cortical spreading depression of Leão*, and takes place in the occipital lobe. I know of two neuro-ophthalmologists who have photographed the vasospasm in the retina during retinal migraine.

One caution: The symptoms of basilar migraine are identical to TIAs, transient ischemic attacks, in the posterior circulation. TIAs are a harbinger of a stroke, even in a young person. I always evaluate these cases thoroughly to rule out the possibility of an impending stroke.

We continue with basilar migraine in Chapter Five in the story **Seven Years of Hell**, but now let's turn our attention to another common and under-recognized cause of migraine.

Migraine Associated with Manic Trait

There's much to be learned from the next story. It takes the "headache is only a symptom" idea a step farther by showing how a benign headache, like migraine, can have a not-so-benign underlying cause. The story also alludes to subsets of underlying causes, and then goes on to show how fundamentally different my approach is from the way it's done today. This difference becomes the subject of Chapters Seven and Eight.

> *Vivacious:* "My last neurologist put me on Topamax. It helped some, but then I couldn't remember things. I had to stop it so I could function at work."

This 42 year-old woman came with a twenty year history of headaches that no doctor could cure. Her MRI was normal. Bloodwork showed no underlying medical problem. The headaches had the character of migraine, and she had them in some form just about every day.

If I only had one word to describe this woman, it would be **Vivacious**. She had a big toothy smile. She was animated and fast-talking. She looked anxious. She was expressive, even a little loud, a bit in-your-face, definitely alive. I sat there wondering, "Could she be a little on the manic side?"

After she gave her story, my first question was three

simple words, "Do you sleep?"

"No." She couldn't initiate sleep. When she eventually did fall asleep, she woke up after two hours and couldn't get back to sleep. So she ran tired all day. As far as I was concerned, she had a subtle form of manic illness until proven otherwise.

The brain chemistry of mania creates a heightened state of vigilance, so intense that a person cannot sleep. The balance between glutamate, an excitatory neurotransmitter, and GABA, an inhibitory neurotransmitter, in the brain seem to be the main problem. There's too much glutamate (excitatory) effect. Depakote corrects this, replacing vigilance with a sense of calm.

I prescribed a modest dose of Depakote with dinner for the next eight days, and asked her to return. It's a reasonably safe and easy way to correct mild forms of the manic trait.

She returned eight days later. She was calm now, and went on to say, "When I take Depakote, I sleep, and when I sleep, I don't get headaches."

After 20 years of headache, we had the answer in only eight days. In one sentence she gave me the pathogenesis.

In just eight days, we learned three important things: First, if I can get her to sleep, she won't have headaches. Second, Depakote is the magic that does just that. Because it's Depakote that gives her a calm feeling inside, I know a third thing: she indeed has a mild form of the manic brain chemistry. We had the answer in only eight days. In one sentence she gave me the pathogenesis.

Depakote can cause weight-gain, so I transitioned her to Lamictal, which is also highly effective for mania, but doesn't cause weight-gain.

Two months later, she returned for her third visit. Her first words: "You know Dr. Smith; I don't think I have to come back here anymore. When I take Lamictal, I sleep, and I told you before, when I sleep I don't get headaches."

Then she said something that sends a chill up my spine every time I think of it.

"For the first time in my life, I know what it's like to feel peace inside. If I had this twenty years ago, I never would have been divorced."

The manic brain chemistry makes a person testy at times. I'm sure that didn't help her marriage.

Headache is never the problem

So the problem wasn't headache. The cure, in this case, came from treating her mania, not the headache. That's what made this a success story.

The more fascinating discovery, as I mentioned earlier, wasn't what finally made her better. It was why the headaches defied a cure for so long in the first place, twenty years for this unfortunate woman. The reason she suffered so long is obvious. All the doctors were treating the wrong thing. Headache was just a symptom of something deeper, the manic trait, that kept her from getting a good night's rest. The fatigue, in turn, activated her migraine. When the volume control on vigilance was turned down with Depakote, she slept like a baby, the headaches resolved and "For the first time in my life, I know what it's like to feel peace inside." The Depakote sweetened up her personality as well. The manic trait, an error in glutamate/GABA chemistry, was the real problem all along. Mania, even in a mild form, may not be so benign. It does make a person energetic, productive and even vivacious; but it can also make a person contentious and make a mess of relationships.

What I learned from this case and others like it is that headache is never the problem. There's always something beneath the surface that causes the headache. Find and correct that and you will have a definitive cure.

Headache is never the problem. There's always something beneath the surface that causes the headache.

Subsets of migraine

This woman's story is an example of another important property of migraine: Migraine is not a single thing. It's composed of distinct groups, what we might call subsets. Each subset activates migraine in a particular way. There are many of these subsets. Each is defined by its unique pathogenesis.

This notion of subsets explains a puzzling property of the medications that we use to prevent migraine: A medication that is very effective for one person may not work at all for another. You can't conclude that just because Depakote worked in this case, it will work in the next. The next case might have basilar artery migraine like *Go-getter* in Chapter Three. She might come back to say, "Depakote only made things worse!" In her case, verapamil will be the answer because her migraine had a different mechanism: stress-adrenaline-vasospasm.

For the sake of clarity, I've simplified this concept of migraine subsets and how they are identified through trials of disease-defining molecules. Using medications this way gets complicated because medications usually have multiple effects. Depakote, for example, may have helped *Vivacious* by either of two effects: its effect on mania or by its anticonvulsant effect on an occult seizure disorder. If a person's headaches improve dramatically on Depakote, and I'm not sure whether it fixed a seizure disorder or mania, then I might do a Tegretol trial. Tegretol has a strong benefit for most forms of epilepsy, but only a weak benefit for mania. A lithium trial can be used in a similar way. Mania will respond to Depakote and lithium. Epilepsy responds to Depakote, but not lithium.

For years we've used Depakote for migraine without knowing why it worked in one person and not in another. It all becomes clear when we realize that Depakote doesn't treat the headache; it's treating the brain chemistry of mania, and that happens to be the underlying cause for many people.

Migraine is not one thing. It's composed of distinct groups. I think of them as subsets of migraine.

The notion of migraine subsets is nothing new. What is new is how we identify them. It doesn't help to pull some trait, like type-A or "prone to stress", out of the air and then do a survey to see if these traits are overrepresented in the migraine population. What I am saying is that the subset must be defined by its pathogenesis. The causes of type-A behavior, as an example, are diverse: mania, worry, anxiety, anger, hyperthyroidism, to name a few. Each responds to its own unique treatment. The comment, "When I take Depakote, I sleep and when I sleep, I don't get headaches." Well, that defines the pathogenesis, doesn't it? Depakote corrects the brain chemistry of mania; it doesn't help the other possible causes of type-A personality.

As you read on, you will see some other migraine subsets.

Worry Headaches

Would you believe that headaches can be caused by worry, or even guilt? Here's how it happens.

No Reason Why: She's sitting on the exam table as I ask, "So, do you have any idea why you get so many headaches?"

With an air of helpless desperation in her voice, she throws her hands up and looks to the sky, "Dr. Smith, I have no idea!"

I turn to her husband, who's sitting on a low stool at her side. "How about you; do you have any ideas?"

"Oh I could tell you in a minute, Doc . . ."

Swiping her hand down through the air at him, she cuts him off in mid-sentence. "Oh, you! You're asleep by the time your head hits the pillow!" she says with more than a little hostility in her voice.

He was about to say that she worries about every little thing. "If she doesn't have anything to worry about, she looks for something. Everything stresses her. She gets all worked up about things that wouldn't faze most people." She doesn't sleep very well, she's tired all the time, and then she gets headaches.

Her headaches went on and on for years. No one could fix them. To her husband, the cause was obvious. Could she really have had no idea why?

One of My Pills: Another woman, this one about thirty, a mother of two young children, had headaches all the time. On her first visit, she surely looked like a worrier to me. She was tired all the time and didn't sleep particularly well. So I gave her a trial of Ambien. This should induce sleep rapidly whether she was worrying or not. "Come back in ten days."

Ten days later she stormed into the office, furious; shaking her finger at me as if I were a naughty little boy. "I took just *one* of your pills, Dr. Smith, and the next thing I knew, I was waking up the next morning. I have no idea what happened that night!"

That one pill (of mine) was diagnostic. She was trying to sleep with her head a half inch off the pillow, listening for things.

When headaches go on and on, and nothing seems to help, worry proves to be the underlying cause most of the time. So why is it so hard to see and so hard to fix? Let me pass along what I've come to understand about worry and suggest an approach that I've used with some success.

When headaches go on and on, and nothing seems to help, worry proves to be the underlying cause most of the time.

Worry is obsessing

Although I'm not what you'd call a worrier, it seems that even

I have the worry mechanism in some primitive form.

> *Sip of Coffee:* One summer I was out in the garage making some drawers with my table saw. I got tired and went into the house for a nap. Fifteen minutes later, I woke up, made a cup of coffee, and went back out to the garage. After working for a few minutes, I turned the saw off and remembered there was a little sip of coffee left in the bottom of the mug. "Darn! Where'd it go?" I searched high and low, getting more frustrated by the minute. Finally I went back into the house, wondering if I'd left it in the kitchen. Not there, either. As I walked back out to the garage, more than a little worked up, I spotted the mug sitting on a stack of wood behind the garage where I had left it. I gulped down the last sip, then, "Ahhhh." relief. Frustration gone, I could relax and get on with what I was doing.

What you're observing in action here is a brain mechanism that's responsible for obsessing. It's a frontal lobe mechanism, carried out by the cortico-striato-thalamo-cortical loop that keeps things going in our head until there is some kind of resolution or closure. The longer it takes to get that closure, the more frustrated a person becomes. Fundamentally then, worry is obsessing.

The strength of this obsessing mechanism varies from person to person. It's genetically determined, so a person is born with a brain that has a strong tendency to worry . . . or not. If we are born with the kind of brain that does not tend to obsess, if our brain does not hold on to concerns, then if we get an upsetting letter during the day, we have upset feelings at that moment, just like anyone else. However, by the end of the day, the thought has slipped out of our head and, chances are, we sleep like a baby. A person who doesn't obsess can't keep an unpleasant thought going in his or her head.

It's the opposite for a person who is born with a worry kind of brain. They can't turn the thought off. It keeps going and going and going until it becomes intrusive, popping up when he or she least wants it, especially when they try to fall asleep. A worrier goes about with this distressing, unsettled feeling all the time. Some things just can't be resolved quickly, so there's always plenty going on up there in the frontal lobe, for which they can't get relief. Just as this frustration kept me searching for the coffee mug, the same feeling makes anyone want to get closure on what's going on in their head. It's just particularly strong in a worrier. And, as I said, it's inborn. Is it any wonder then that worriers have problems with sleep?

I don't mean to suggest the worry trait is entirely genetic. If, for example, a family puts the caretaker responsibility onto a child born with a tendency to worry, that trait might easily be intensified. Another family might even decondition worry, simply by the way it functions. Later we'll see how nurture can be used to moderate this trait, which is part of a person's genetic nature.

Several neurotransmitters operate the worry circuit. The most important effect seems to come from serotonin. Drugs like amitriptyline and Prozac increase serotonin in this circuit, decrease worry, and make a person more carefree.

Don't you wonder why we have a circuit and chemistry to make us obsess? I think it's because someone who *doesn't* worry has a disadvantage in a way, because some things just need to be worried about. We need this circuit to make us attend to a threat, not ignore it. Ignore a threat and bad things might happen.

The Neanderthals didn't have much of a frontal lobe; we know that from the anatomy of their skull. So they probably didn't have much of a worry circuit, either. I wonder if that's why they went extinct. They didn't worry enough about things that needed to be worried about. The Neanderthals were driven to extinction when Cro-Magnon man, the first humans, appeared. We know that our Cro-Magnon ancestors had big frontal lobes. They must have had a greater capacity to worry about things and that made them take action against any threat. Worry seems to have survival value.

Fundamentally, worry is obsessing. To understand the pathogenesis of worry headaches, we must understand how worry works.

How worry works

Worry activates migraine in three ways. To understand the pathogenesis of worry headaches, it helps to understand first how worry works.

Worry wears you out: First, a person who tends to worry or obsess about things has a great deal going on all the time in that frontal lobe circuit of theirs. So their brain is awfully busy keeping track of all the things they need to worry about, that doesn't happen so much in the brain of a person who does not worry.

> *The Simple of It:* One morning I was at the computer, writing, when a patient called with side effects from two

medications. Both are safe and generally well tolerated. She came as a multiple sclerosis (MS) suspect with recurrent pain beginning six years earlier that had become severe over the few days before I saw her. Workup to date had shown no MS. I suspected a herpesvirus was causing the pain and prescribed two medications. The essence of her call was "I can't take Neurontin. It makes me drowsy. Valtrex made me nauseated."

Instead, she went on with details, many details, what seemed like irrelevant details, but never mentioned the important thing: Did they help the pain? The clock was ticking, I needed to get back to what I was doing, and I was getting worn out with so much information about side effects and no mention about what I needed to know. So I interrupted; something that's hard for me to do. "Well, the simple of it . . . We think that a herpesvirus is causing the pain. Are you any better after the few doses of Valtrex? She gave me a definite "Yes."

"So it looks like herpesvirus, not MS is causing these symptoms. Don't take any more medication. If the nausea is gone by noon, it's probably the Valtrex. If it continues after Valtrex is out of your system, it's something else. Give me a call tomorrow and let me know what happened." End of phone call.

When I hung up, it felt as if I needed a nap and a cup of coffee. What goes through *my* head all day? It's much simpler. Even so, my brain gets tired by the end of the day. I can't imagine what it's like for *her* brain. She just can't stop all that "busy-ness" going on up there. All the things that a worrier worries about, they go on and on all the time. That would wear anybody out.

Strong unpleasant emotions: The second thing about worry that tends to activate headache is the strong, unpleasant emotions that the worry generates. Usually, when a person worries, it's about some threat, something unpleasant. So it may provoke anxiety or grieving or anger or other distressing emotion. Strong emotions like this kick up adrenaline, make it hard to sleep and activate headache. It isn't that the worrier has strong emotions. Who doesn't? The problem is that the obsessing won't let go, so the emotions just don't stop.

Lack of restorative sleep: Finally, worriers often have a hard time getting restorative sleep. The difference between a person who worries and a person who doesn't is especially evident when stress rears its ugly head. For someone who doesn't worry, sleep is an escape, a welcome respite from an upsetting day, a time to recharge the brain and be in better shape to handle the stress in the morning. Its like going into a room and locking the door. "There, I'm safe. Nothing can harm me now."

For a worrier it's different; when it's time to sleep, the thoughts keep repeating. "I can't shut my brain off." All the things running through a worrier's mind during the day won't quit. They become uncontrollably intrusive. So they fall asleep watching TV or listening to audio books, which pulls their attention away from what's running in their cortico-striato-thalamo-cortical loop.

Even when someone who worries does fall asleep quickly and sleeps through the night, one might hear, "I can sleep eight hours, but I still wake up tired." "I'm a light sleeper. Any little noise wakes me up." A formal sleep study explains why. We typically see a high arousal index in individuals who tend to worry. This means that the person flips between sleep states every few minutes. They don't stay in a particular stage of sleep for the ten or twenty minutes it takes for that stage of sleep to regenerate the chemistry of the brain. One lady with considerable insight commented, "It's as if I'm worrying in my sleep." However this may happen, one thing is clear: A person needs to stay in each stage of sleep for a length of time if sleep is to be restorative and refreshing.

> **Worry wears us out. It creates strong, unpleasant emotions and interferes with the sleep we need to recover**

In *Fibromyalgia and Restorative Sleep* I suggested that restorative sleep somehow replenishes the chemistry of the brain, especially the neurotransmitters that allow us to think and learn and remember. Sleep that regenerates our brain this way is essential to the circuits that control pain. When for any reason we do not get good sleep, the continual depletion of brain chemistry creates a state of chronic pain. In some people this expresses itself as headache, in others as fibromyalgia and in still others as both.

Saying it differently, restorative sleep is a must. I tell my patients that I have discovered a fundamental rule of the universe, something like $e = mc^2$. My rule is this: "If you don't get restorative sleep, you'll never get rid of your headaches."

I never could appreciate how depleting worry is until I saw one of my patients agonize over an important decision. Like so many decisions in life, this one had no clear answer. A few days on an SSRI, and she gracefully made the decision with ease.

Recognizing worry

One of the first questions I hear is, "Okay, so I worry too much. How do I fix it?" Before we can go there, we need to understand how to recognize worry and how it tends to play out in life.

> *12-year-old:* I asked a twelve-year-old girl, "Do you worry about things?"
>
> Her answer: "No. I don't worry at all. I'm as laid-back as they come." Mom nodded her head in agreement. She looked like a worrier to me: pleasant, in control, unusually articulate, anything but carefree.
>
> "Suppose you got a C-?"
>
> A startle came to her face, pupils dilated, eyes wide open. I thought, "I'm not seeing laid-back now. Another kid might just say, 'I got a C- . . . So what?' This one's a worrier all right."

The story a worrier tells might be anything. It might come from a young boy, an old woman, or anything in between. I can't say that there is one story that's characteristic of worry. The stories vary as much as the individuals who live them out. It might be the story of an executive who just can't get rid of his headaches or a school-age boy or girl who is outstanding in every way, but always has a headache. It might come from an overcommitted mother of five; just about anything you might imagine.

If it's hard to recognize worry from the story, then it's easy to recognize worry by how the story is told. The stories always contain markers for worry. Like a beacon, they allow you to hone-in on the trait, even when the person says, "Me? I'm not a worrier."

The first tip-off is the appearance of the person who tells the story. A worrier typically seems well put together, well groomed, pleasant, even to the point of being gracious. They may even have an air of peace about them; but if he or she is emotionally distressed, there's a giveaway: it's the face of worry, a twisted wrinkle between the eyebrows and a kind of tension in the mouth. It's hard to put into words, so I won't even try. The best way to see it is to look at the face of a person you know is a worrier. They all seem to have it.

The face of worry is one of the best markers. Another is the caregiver. Some of the most compassionate people I know come out of this profile.

The second clue is how the story is told. It's told in a way that's distinct from other personality styles. Almost invariably, we hear strong themes of responsibility and care-giving accompanied by many concerns about many things. A worrier is quite distressed by things that wouldn't bother most people. "My husband's uncle had a heart attack a month ago. He's okay now, but I'm concerned about the future." I'm thinking, "Gee, that wouldn't bother me."

So we hear what-ifs that seem a little odd, because the thoughts wouldn't even pass through the head of the average person, let alone be a source of concern. In men it often goes like this:

> *Worst Case Scenario:* "Okay, Doc, what's the worst case scenario here."
>
> "Well, the worst case scenario for me is that I get killed in a motor vehicle accident on my way home tonight. I don't want you thinking about the worst case. You need to be thinking about the most likely scenarios; plan for them."

The worrier can be a little intimidating when we discuss the diagnosis.

> *Intimidating:* "So why do you think I'm getting all these headaches?"
>
> "I think you're just wearing yourself out trying to take care of everybody. You worry too much, and that tires your brain out. The things you worry about create a lot of stress, and then you can't sleep. I'd like to get a scan and some bloodwork, just to be sure there's no serious problem."
>
> "Oh my God! You think I have a tumor? Will I need surgery? Could it be cancer?"

Can you see what I mean about this innate tendency to focus on the unlikely, at the expense of what the person really needs to be thinking about? What I was trying to say is that the problem is the worry and all that goes along with it. That's what we need to be thinking about right now. The tests are just to be sure that we don't miss anything serious. That's what I tried to say, but somehow what I said got reinterpreted. Getting a scan would be reassuring, comforting to most people, but the worrier made the message into something to worry about.

Reinterpretation of what we hear is a curious phenomenon. Often called *confirmation bias*, it's a form of perceptual distortion in which a person reinterprets what is said, events of the past or any event for that matter, to align with their own beliefs. It's one reason why we don't learn new things. It's also a window into the mind of the person. I even have an entertaining story about it, but all this is beyond what we're discussing here.

If you think of worry as obsessing, you can see how it creates a variety of troublesome feelings. Obsess about the loss of a loved one, and you become depressed. Obsess about money, and you might look anxious. The overbearing conscience that goes along with this trait may make it hard for the worrier to forgive himself for something he's done. "I promised that I would always watch over her. Now look at me. She has to take care of me." To make it worse, the anguish never ends.

There is a kind of vigilance associated with worry, although the mechanism is different from that of mania. The vigilance of mania is due to excitatory brain chemistry. Worry vigilance is a consequence of obsessing. Vigilance is a natural state of alertness that keeps us focused on life's perils. Vigilance explains the "what ifs" and the concern about worst case scenarios so characteristic of those who worry.

Another marker for a person who worries is an inordinate concern about possible harmful side effects of medication. "I don't want pills." The concerns seem to be blown way out of proportion to the reality, which is something that worriers tend to do. So, many worriers seldom or never take medication. Some even speak badly of the physician who prescribes them. It seems like it's only a worrier who would take the time to read that detailed printout of side effects we get from the pharmacist. "I was afraid to take that pill you prescribed, Dr. Smith. Did you know it can actually *cause* a headache?" Caution is a trait that is overrepresented in this personality profile.

Unusual sensitivity to medications is yet another earmark of worry. "When I take just a quarter tablet of aspirin, I'm in a coma for two days." "Odd," I thought. "She doesn't have an aspirin allergy. How could such a low dose do this?"

A need for perfection often accompanies worry. A perfectionist looks at a messy desk and gets stressed. Every little thing is seen as important and must be brought to closure. Another person might just address two or three of the most important things on the desk and, with his arm, brush the rest onto the floor, and go home satisfied, I might add.

The perfectionist often has a hard time telling the difference between what's important and what isn't important. Everything is important. To say it a different way, worriers often lack *salience* determination.

If we think of worry as obsessing, it's easy to see how vigilance, perfectionism, obsessive-compulsive disorder and other repetitive behaviors might be more common in those who worry. Benign tic disorder is another.

In summary then, several signs help identify the worrier. Perfectionism, a strong need for completion, what you might call closure, and what seems to be a higher than average need for control are markers for worry. They easily become over-programmed and exhaust themselves, getting everything done. So look for the what ifs, rejection of medications, and an uncommon sensitivity to medications and anxiety. When you hear, "It all falls on me." that's the language of responsibility, another marker. If the person has headaches that no one can cure, think worry.

The face of worry is one of the best markers. Another is recognizing the caregiver. Some of the most compassionate people I know come out of this profile.

The list goes on, but that's enough for now.

How worry plays out in life

Life seems to unfold in a particular way according to the kind of person we are. As someone who doesn't worry, I've lived out the glory and the grief of having that trait. Life plays out differently for the one who worries.

> *Non-organic Seizures:* Not long after opening my practice, I got a call from a physician in an outlying community. He had a woman in the hospital who was having one seizure after another, despite very high doses of anticonvulsants. He called to transfer her care to the University.
>
> Shortly after she arrived, I walked into her room and there she was having a generalized seizure. The first thing I do when a person is seizing is to lift their eyelids to see what their eyes are doing. She was looking around the room with the saccadic eye movements of a person who is fully awake. So I knew that she was not having an electrical seizure; clearly her seizures were non-organic.

Non-organic means that the person does not have a physical

problem causing the symptom. In this case, she was not having electrical seizure activity. So it's no wonder that the anti-epileptic medications didn't work. Whether or not the shaking is intentional or caused by the dark subconscious is a matter of debate. That's not the important question here.

By now I know you're saying to yourself, "The more fascinating question is *why* she was having non-organic seizures." Good question.

> As the seizure ended, she opened her eyes. In the gentlest voice that I could muster, I said that I could see that these were not electrical seizures. "Usually this kind of seizure is caused by some emotional stress. Pain is a better word than stress, not a pain in your body; it's a pain in your heart." We connected instantly. She knew what I was talking about.
>
> She began by telling me about life at home. She was taking care of her mother-in-law with Alzheimer's disease. "I couldn't bear to see her in a nursing home." She planned to take care of her to the bitter end. On top of that, she had overwhelming family responsibilities. True to form, she was a lovely, gracious human being, a caregiver and a worrier for sure.
>
> I spoke with the family, pointing out the heavy burden on her shoulders, to which, in good conscience, she just could not allow herself to say "No." They understood immediately. She was discharged after a few days, off medication, free of seizures. Mother-in-law was put into a nursing home.
>
> Once or twice a year after that, I would hear a knock on my office door. It would open and in popped her head with a big smile. "I just want you to know, Dr. Smith - I'm doing fine. No seizures."

Too much responsibility, more care-giving than is humanly possible, an over-programmed life, whatever you want to call it, it's a common downfall of the worrier.

Too much responsibility, more care-giving than is humanly possible, an over-programmed life, whatever you want to call it, it's a common downfall of the worrier.

One reason life plays out differently is that a person who worries sees things differently.

> *Feet Kicked Up:* "I get headaches all the time, usually in the left eye. Every week or two they turn into

a migraine, but even on my good days, I have a headache of some form. Light seemed to trigger the one I had two weeks ago. Everything is going well. There's just no reason why I should be getting these headaches now."

"How's your sleep?" I asked.

"I sleep okay."

"Do you feel refreshed in the morning?"

"Never . . . I'm tired all the time."

"Do you worry about things?"

"No more than anybody else."

In her forties, she's an executive in a midsized corporation, highly responsible and highly effective. Worry was written all over her face. She had the telltale signs all right.

"How are things at home?"

"I get home and make supper, and then I do the dishes and clean up the kitchen. Everybody's out in the living room watching TV. My husband's out there with his feet kicked up. He doesn't even help. All the responsibility falls on me."

Another worry theme: responsibility. A better night's sleep might help. I offer her Ambien.

"I'd like to know if a good night's sleep helps your fatigue and the headaches."

She declines. "I don't take medications. I don't think it's good to put all of those chemicals into your body." So we proceed with an MRI of the head and some bloodwork and she returns two weeks later with her husband. The studies are normal.

Looking at her husband, I ask, "Do you have any idea why she gets so many headaches?"

"I tell her all the time, Doc. She's a worrywart. Everything's gotta be perfect. If somebody's late or something's out of place, she's upset. Then she gets a headache."

Then he spontaneously offered a different point of view of his wife's feet-kicked-up comment. "Let me tell you how it goes. After supper, I'll be in the living room with the kids, and she's in the kitchen doing the dishes or some other thing. I tell her, 'Don't worry about the dishes,

Honey. They're not important. I want you out here with us. I just want to put my arm around you.'"

I thought, "What's more important here, the dishes or spending some time with her family?" She was so uncomfortable when the kitchen was not in order that she couldn't even relax enough to enjoy her family. Then a perceptual distortion appears. She feels taken advantage of when everyone else doesn't follow her high expectations. She puts her burdens onto her loved ones because that's just the way she sees things. Her expectations even create a bit of a rift with her husband, which is another problem.

It seemed to me that she had a perceptual distortion going on.

His comment made good sense to me. I even wondered, "Suppose she divorced her husband, gave the kids away, and moved to Chicago. I'll bet that after a year she'll be in the same kind of situation. That's what's trying to happen."

What makes this story so important is the way my patient saw things, her perceptions, and how they differed so from those of her husband. I'm sure it wasn't true, but it almost seemed as if order and completion were more important than having time with her loved ones.

If a worrier trips up in the perception department, then it may also be true that a greater awareness of perceptions might be an effective source of healing. Just as a person with a foot drop tends to trip on his toe, being mindful of it prevents the stumbling. In this case, my patient might have said, "You know Honey, I think you've got something there. I really *would* like to be with you and the kids. How about this: You help me with the dishes. The kids make their lunches. In twenty minutes we could be watching TV together, and you can put your arm around me all evening."

Not only is worry common, it's hard to change. That makes worry a likely cause of headaches that no one seems able to fix.

In a moment, I will continue with non-medication approaches, beginning with a story that shows the critical importance of this perceptual change. Before we consider how to make worry better without pills, let me try to explain why it's so hard to fix.

A tough nut to crack

Not only is worry common, it's hard to change. That makes worry a likely cause of headaches that go on and on, headaches that no one seems able to fix. So when I see a person for long-standing headaches that no one can cure, one of the first things that comes to mind is, "Could this be some form of benign headache, perhaps migraine, driven by a tendency to worry?"

Manic illness, bipolar disorder, depression, anxiety, and worry all respond to medications. Even when a medication does work, a worrier will often stop taking the medication out of concern for weight gain or other side effect. So, treating worry isn't the easiest thing in the world. That's one reason the headaches are so hard to fix. Worry, however, is one trait that always needs something more than just a medication. This is the bad news.

The good news is that non-medication approaches can be quite effective. Which leads to more bad news: If you worry, it may take more than just a pill to make the worry go away. It takes effort, some emotional work and, like growing a prized flower in your garden, it takes time. Growing as a person and bettering ourselves is something we all must do in life. It's easy to spot the person who hasn't.

The Wright Brother's principle: Before we jump into what may prove to be a long journey of treatment, it's nice to know if worry is indeed the culprit. So I often begin with a trial of medications known to be effective for worry, just to be sure the headaches respond when we turn the volume control down on worry. Let me say it this way.

Imagine you are one of the Wright Brothers. You finally get your aircraft to stay aloft for twelve seconds. You know now that you are *capable* of flight. You're one step ahead; you've got the lift principle working. Now you need some control surfaces, so you can steer the aircraft, and then a better engine.

In the same way, if the headaches resolve with a medication for worry, even for a week or two, then we know we're on the right track. The headache isn't neuralgia, a brain tumor or something else we might have missed. We know that the person is capable of living headache-free, capable of flying in a sense. We can celebrate and move on to the next step. I call this the Wright Brothers' principle.

On the other hand, if treatment with medications for worry does not help, then we'd better think again. We'd better consider other possibilities before we spend a year trying to manage worry with non-medication methods. Maybe the problem isn't worry. The medication failure suggests that a non-medication approach may not work, either. The Wright Brothers may never have succeeded if they had worked on other details of their aircraft without first getting the thing to stay in the air.

When I suspect worry is the activator of a person's migraine, and the patient agrees to a medication trial, I may offer a *tricyclic* or *SSRI* trial for two weeks. These medications upregulate serotonin, downregulate worry, and make a person more carefree. If it takes a long time to fall asleep, we might trial Ambien, which rapidly turns on the sleep switch without tranquilizing the person.

Giddy: Imagine a twelve-year-old girl, a total love of a person, very mindful of not hurting anyone's feelings, who has a headache every day. We wonder, "Is this just poor sleep and a susceptibility to worry or something more serious?" That wasn't the only concern. Whatever the cause, even though she wasn't missing school, every day the headache made life difficult, less enjoyable.

With the Wright Brothers' principle in mind, I suggested a 10 day trial of low dose *doxepin*, "for diagnostic purposes."

Ten days later Mom called. "I can't believe it. From the day after the first dose she's had no headache at all for 10 days. She was having them every day. I gave her the pill at dinnertime, and a few hours later she even seemed a little giddy. There she was: lighthearted, not the serious person she usually is. It was good to see her joking around for a change."

In just 10 days, the Wright Brothers' principle had told us what we needed to know. We knew that she was capable of being completely free of headache.

The medication lost its benefit after two weeks. Another doctor increased the dose by ten times. There were side effects, and she had a hard time coming off the medication, even with a very slow taper. The other doctor was using doxepin for treatment. I was using it for diagnosis.

In just 10 days, the Wright Brothers' principle had told us what we needed to know: First, the fact that she was headache-free for 10 days meant that there was no serious underlying problem, no brain tumor. We knew that she was capable of being completely free of headache.

Second, because a low dose of doxepin was so successful, we knew that worry, the serotonin brain chemistry and maybe even a bit of depression, was the fundamental problem. So the medication pointed our nose to the answer. Her strong favorable response left us reasonably certain that worry was the problem. The diagnosis had been confirmed with a *disease-defining molecule*.

The problem with pills: Knowing that worry is behind the headaches, we might use medications at first, but with time and some effort, there's a good chance that non-medication approaches will obviate the need for a pill. One advantage of non-medication approaches is that they leave a person adaptive. If we treat worry with a pill, then a person becomes carefree all the time. Who wants that? With non-medication approaches, a person can worry about things that need to be worried about and be carefree when they just want to have fun, and of course, no weight gain from medications.

Three Women: It's interesting to see what happens when a medication trial strongly supports worry as the primary problem. Imagine three women with headaches that go away on worry medications. Then what happens? I've seen it go three different ways.

One might return to say, "Dr. Smith, I told you when I came, 'I'm looking for a fix.' On Ambien and Paxil, I sleep much better, I'm not tired all the time, and the headaches go away. Just give me my pills, and I'll be out of your hair." The problem here is that she'll be eighty years old and still fumbling around in her pocket for the pills.

Another might say, "Well, now I know how all this works. Yes, I worry too much. I totally understand what you're saying, but I don't like putting these chemicals into my body." So she stops the medications and then goes back to where she was, sleepless and tired all the time with headaches. At least now we know the reason why.

A third woman, if I ever see her again, might return in a year or two and say "You know I still have the Ambien and Paxil in my medicine cabinet. Once in a while I use them, but *I really don't need them any more.*" What she's done is to find non-medication ways to decondition worry and obsessing. It may have taken a while, but she's done her homework. That's at the heart of becoming well, and that's what I strongly recommend.

When it's clear that obsessing is at the heart of the problem, I always recommend non-medication approaches

In those who seem to worry, a medication trial can be a helpful diagnostic tool, even if it's only for a week. If we can turn worry down for a week with a pill and the headaches get better, then it's clear what we have to work on. I go on to explain that I use pills differently, not only for treatment. Many are *diagnostic molecules* or, if you prefer, *disease-defining molecules.*

I'm not always stuck, though, when a person flat-out refuses medication. Often the trait is so strong that patient and doctor alike are certain that it's worry from the get-go. Then we might launch right into non-medication approaches.

Non-medication approaches

With or without a medication trial, when it's clear that the obsessing trait is at the heart of the problem, I always recommend non-medication approaches to treatment. There are a number of these, and they are often used along with medication for worry. That's a topic for another book. Success depends on the severity of the worry, the environment and the person. Here's an introduction.

A change in perceptions: Amid the complexities of worry and its treatment, one thing must occur if a worrier is ever to be well.

> *Conversion Experience:* A woman about sixty came for evaluation of her vision. She was one of those lovely human beings who one could easily see as a person susceptible to worry, no question about it. Feelings transpersonalize and the feeling I got from her was one of peace, not the angst so characteristic of worry. I couldn't resist saying, "Before we go on . . . you know something's really bothering me. You have all the markers of a person who worries about things, but you don't seem to be bothered by little things, the way a worrier often is."
>
> "Oh, I used to be a terrible worrier. Every little thing stressed me. If my husband was late or someone wasn't doing their job, if things weren't just so, I'd get terribly upset, and then I'd get a headache. I don't do that anymore."
>
> "That's fascinating. Don't leave me hanging. What brought the change?"
>
> A sad look came to her face. "It all changed when we found that my son had leukemia . . . That taught me what was important in life and what didn't matter at all. The little things that used to get me so upset; it doesn't bother me anymore. It's not important."

What happened to this woman was neither pill nor psychotherapy. It was more like a religious conversion experience than anything else I can think of. Her heart-wrenching experience, the possible loss of her son, brought about an immediate and dramatic change in the way she saw things and how she made sense out of the events of life. Now when her husband is late, she isn't upset or angry. The thought that comes to her head is, "Oh, that's not important." That was the thought that replaced the old thoughts that made her upset. This new way of seeing things did just the opposite. It was calming.

One might say that her son's illness was perceptual psychotherapy. I see it as a dramatic change in the spirit in which she lived her life. In the deepest sense, it was a turnaround at the spiritual level of her existence.

If it's true that worry drives the headache, and also true that perceptions drive the worry, then without a change in how we see things, there may be no end in sight to the headaches. This explains why it's so tough to fix headache in a person who worries, even with medication. Perceptions are simply hard to change.

A change in preoccupation: You might say that this woman was still obsessive. It's just that there was a change in what she obsessed about. Before the leukemia, she obsessed about "every little thing." After, her obsession was "Oh, that's not important." Obsess about one thing, and it makes you anxious or angry. Obsess about something else, and it gives you hope and may even lead you to fix whatever you're worried about. If you obsess about the dishes and "It all falls on me." then how could a person be anything but angry. On the other hand, obsess about enjoying life and spending time with loved ones, including your husband who just wants to put his arm around you, and you feel better inside. You might even obsess about a loving way to get the rest of the family to help. The situation is the same. It's just seen differently. There's more than one way to look at any situation in life, and they're not equally healthy.

Acquiring more healthy ways to see things, growing in this way, is something we all must do. One thing is for sure: There's no guarantee that life will be flawless. In fact, most of us will encounter a calamity at some time in life. One way of seeing things might be the start of a spiral downward, at a time when those about us need just the opposite. With a different perception, we could become the Rock of Gibraltar, at a time when that's what our loved ones need the most.

The best predictor: The best way to know if a person will make a change like this is whether the worry trait is *ego-syntonic*

Without a change in how we see things, there may be no end in sight to the headaches.

or *ego-alien*. Consider smoking, for example. If a person says, "Doc, I'm a smoker. That's just me." Smoking is ego-syntonic for this person. He sees smoking as part of his natural self, so he's not likely to change.

On the other hand, if a person says, "I've tried to quit tobacco three times and never succeeded. I hate smoking. I worry about cancer. I can't afford it. But I just can't seem to quit." This person will eventually quit because he sees smoking as ego-alien. Smoking is something he doesn't like about himself. Sooner or later, the cigarettes will go.

It's the same with worry. If a person says, "I'm just a natural-born worrier. That's just the way I am." It's not likely to change. When your daughter goes out for a ride on her bike, and you're thinking, "Oh my God . . . What if she has an accident? . . . What if she's hit by a car? . . . What if she's abducted?" Then you say to yourself, "Wait a minute. It's not healthy to think that way." This is the person who will change, no matter how hard it is to make that change. Being mindful of our perceptions, how we see things, and asking ourselves, "Is it healthy to think this way?" is one of the best signs of a healthy mind.

I find that any disorder, if it's driven by worry, is hard to treat. Headaches, depression, anxiety, when they occur in a worrier, are often refractory to treatment. It's important in these cases to realize that the greater problem isn't the headache or the depression or the anxiety. It's the obsessing that needs treatment more than anything else. What makes worry so hard to fix isn't just that it's an inborn, hard-wired trait. It's fed by a person's perceptions, one more thing that resists change. It's ironic that stubborn problems like this are so common in individuals who, as a rule, are such nice people.

Obsessing and perceptions are two things that go on inside a person's head. You might guess that I don't think much of exercise or acupuncture or herbal remedies as a cure for worry. They're all external. If you want to worry less, what happens inside your head is so much more important than anything that comes from the outside.

> **If you want to worry less, what happens inside your head is so much more important than anything that comes from the outside.**

Headaches in a Young Person

Headaches in children and young adults can be a challenge. Many of the medications we use in adults are not FDA approved for children, young people tend to be more sensitive to medications and, when it comes to psychoactive medications, children are at risk for depression and suicide. So medication trials in this group are part of the challenge.

On the other hand, these trials are very important. Starting out at a young age with a misdiagnosis has consequences. One reason headaches in a young person are such a challenge is that they often prove to be a chronic form of migraine driven by worry. Again, we're facing a tough nut to crack.

Out of Africa: A 14-year-old boy came with Mom for headaches. He's a really nice fellow, the kind of boy that makes me feel like saying, "Come on home and be my son." He has a headache every day, but he pushes through them. He doesn't miss any school, but I can see that they take a lot out of him. He has pain in his neck muscles. He's sensitive to light. Sometimes he has nausea. I'm not sure whether to call them tension-type headache or chronic daily migraine or mixed pattern headache. Whatever we call them, he has them every day and his MRI scan shows no serious underlying cause.

I've heard these cases referred to as "a neurologist's nightmare." They're hard to fix. We give them a tricyclic at bedtime and about half the time they get better. Often though, nothing we do seems to help. I heard one renowned pediatric neurologist say, "I send them straight to psychiatry."

I saw this young man from time to time over eight months and, to no surprise, nothing I did helped. Every time we tried something, he came back saying, "Yeah, it helped some." Really, Mom and I agreed, he was just being nice to me. Nothing really helped.

He returned for a follow-up appointment in April. His first words were, "Dr. Smith, do you think I can go to Africa this summer?"

I'm thinking, "N-n-n-no! The last thing you want to do is go to Africa. The airplane trip alone will cause a whopper of a headache. Then there's the heat. You won't have any doctor over there to take care of you. You'll be miserable."

Before I could get any of this out, he went on, ". . . because, you remember; you took care of my sister, and

One reason headaches in a young person are such a challenge is that they often prove to be a chronic form of migraine driven by worry.

she didn't have any headaches the summer she was in Africa."

He was much too kind to say the truth: "Remember, you couldn't fix her headaches either."

An image of his sister flashed into my mind. Yes, I remember. The words mature and gracious came to mind. She came out of the same mold.

I said, "Go!"

The next time I saw him was in October, six months later. He had been to Africa and, like his sister, had no headaches. Now, after a month back in school, the headaches were back. "Curious," I thought.

"What did you do in Africa?" I still get a lump in my throat every time I think of what he said.

"We're missionaries. We build homes for people who need them."

I had an image of my young patient waking up in the morning, having some breakfast, pounding some nails through the day, coming back for dinner, having some fellowship with his friends and going to bed for a sound night's sleep.

Just then, his mom chimes in, "You should see him at home. He comes home from school, goes straight upstairs to study, comes down for supper, and then back upstairs to finish all his homework. It doesn't matter how long it takes. He doesn't go to bed until it's finished. You never have to tell him a thing. He's a good kid."

I thought, "Just like his sister."

By now you surely can recognize that this young fellow worries, and the worry activates his inherited susceptibility to migraine. The tip-off: the patient is exceedingly pleasant. He's likable. That's a bad sign. He's also a person who is unusually responsible, a caregiver, and someone who has a strong sense of right and wrong, a conscience, even guilt. It's the worry-obsessing part of the brain that makes a person this way. It's inborn and it runs in families.

So we're a step ahead of the renowned specialist who would have sent him to psychiatry' but where do we go from here? Is there any way to help, beyond taking medication?

The summer in Africa was another application of the Wright

Brothers principle. It proved that he is capable of being headache-free, and even doing it without a pill.

Simplify: The *Out of Africa* story says that if we simply transplant a worrier into an environment that doesn't provoke worry, one that is simple and less demanding, then we can quickly improve how the person feels. I think this is a commentary on our culture, which fosters high achievement and tends to over-program life. I see young people who go to school all day and then get driven around to swimming lessons, music lessons etc. Even going for a swim becomes work. Why not just go for a swim with the kids and have some fun? Let them develop their own interests. I'm not talking about video games, cell phones, and TV here. For the most part, I think they're a waste of time for anybody.

The more complex and the more demanding the environment, the more a worrier has to think about. Anyone else would just let it go and lose track of things; but the person who worries is responsible to the extreme. He keeps track of it all, then adds to that a responsibility for all the things that everyone else has lost track of.

If you worry, simpler is better.

> Not only do we need to simplify our environment; we need to simplify our mind as well.

Salience: Not only do we need to simplify our environment; we need to simplify our mind as well. If there is anything a worrier needs to obsess about, it's the word salient. Becoming aware that too much is going on up there and asking, "What's important here?" is a first step. Understanding that some things are important and others are not is one way to exclude all those intrusive thoughts.

———

I'm so glad this young fellow didn't give me a chance to say, "N-n-n-no! . . . Don't go!" He demonstrated another application of the Wright Brothers' principle, and gave me a good lesson on how worry works.

Chapter Four

Serious Headaches

Serious headaches show that we pay a high price for not looking into underlying cause.

Serious headaches, fortunately, are not common. So it's easy to forgo a thorough evaluation. After all, chances are in your favor that the evaluation will find nothing wrong. Nonetheless, the possibility of a serious underlying cause is a source of concern. "Could this be a brain tumor?" "Do I have an aneurysm?" All too often the patient seems more concerned than the doctor.

Occult Seizure Disorder

Years ago I developed an interest in horseback riding, an interest more than a skill. Before long I wanted to ride through the countryside and found a farm where I could do just that. Galloping through the countryside on horseback is a magnificent, exhilarating experience. The memory always brings a smile to my face.

> *Special Ed:* At the end of the first day riding, I was in the farmhouse paying the bill when the woman who owned the farm looked at my check and said, "Oh, you're a neurologist. My son gets terrible migraine headaches. They've put him in special ed." Then she looked at me and added, "Behavior problems."
>
> "Migraine with a change in behavior could be a sign of epilepsy. He should be evaluated."
>
> "Oh, he's never had a seizure." Nevertheless, she made an appointment. On his first visit, the boy said that sometimes he smelled something burning, not a smell he could recognize. "Funny, nobody else ever smelled it." He

was describing an *uncinate aura*, a symptom of temporal lobe epilepsy. Right then I ordered an EEG and a scan.

Before he had the tests, I was back at the farm, riding. I was paying the bill when Mom mentioned that the boy had one of those bad migraine headaches again that morning. I saw him lying on the couch in the next room. "How are you doing, old fellow?"

"I feel okay."

I went back to pay the bill. A minute or two later we hear, "Thud!" I ran into the room next door and saw the boy on the floor having a generalized convulsion, his first ever, fortuitously witnessed by a neurologist.

His EEG confirmed temporal lobe epilepsy. The MRI scan was normal. I started him on Tegretol, his headaches stopped, the behavioral problems vanished and he returned to regular classes. A few years later, the headaches and behavior came back. A growth spurt had caused his Tegretol blood level to drop, so I increased the dose, and he went right back to normal. He turned out to be a fine young man and eventually assumed management of the farm.

Migraine and Migrainous Headache

In Chapter 3 we saw that migraine can look like other things: eyestrain, "my normal headaches" and, yes, even sinus headaches. I called this phenomenon masquerade migraine.

The young man here shows that other things can look just like migraine.

The young man here shows that the opposite can also happen: other things can look just like migraine. In this case, temporal lobe epilepsy was the underlying cause of his headaches and change in behavior. I use the term "migrainous headache" to say that the headache appears to be migraine, but is not, or may not be migraine in the true sense. I use the term migrainous to mean migraine-like, when I want to leave open the possibility that there may be a potentially serious underlying cause. When I'm sure it's migraine and not caused by a tumor or something like that, I call the headache migraine, rather than migrainous headache.

We can avoid some serious errors in diagnosis if we keep in mind that migraine can look like other things, and other things can look like migraine. You might be saying to yourself, "Okay, makes sense. Then what are we calling migraine in the true sense? What's the definition?" To answer that, let's go back to basics.

Circular reasoning: When a person walks in the door with headaches on one side, nausea and sensitivity to light, one question pops into mind: "Is it migraine or something else?" You can't just say, "If it looks like a duck, walks like a duck and quacks like a duck . . . then it's a duck."

Peepers: I know something about ducks. I grew up in Trenton, New Jersey, just a mile from the state fairgrounds. One day as a young boy, I came home from the fair with a two week-old duckling in my pocket. Peepers and I, we were close. We spent a lot of time together.

Peepers didn't follow the other ducks around, the way ducks do. He followed me, and even seemed to take an interest in whatever I was doing. When I came home from school, he'd spot me, and come flying down the driveway, and land in my arms. Then he'd nuzzle his neck against mine like a long lost friend.

I might be sitting on the back steps, lost in thought when, all of a sudden, I'd feel him jump into my lap. He wanted me to pet him. We even have a picture of me sitting in a tree with Peepers in my arms.

In the summer we had a big washtub in the yard full of water. When I wasn't in it, we'd always find some of our ducks in there swimming around. We couldn't keep them out. Not Peepers. He didn't like to be in water. If you put him in, he'd jump right out.

Peepers looked, walked and quacked like a duck, but he was clearly something more than just a duck. Like many of the creatures we live with these days, he had become humanized. He looked like a duck, but he didn't act like one. He thought I was his mother and got an imprint from me, so he behaved more like a person than a duck. Anyone could tell, "This is no ordinary duck." He had a duck body, but in his head he thought he was a person.

Even though a headache looks like migraine and meets the definition, it doesn't mean that migraine is the entire story.

Here's the point: Even though a headache looks like migraine and meets the definition, it doesn't mean that migraine is the entire story. I've seen headaches that look just like migraine, fit the International Headache Society's (IHS) definition perfectly, but disappeared when the seizure disorder, meningioma, leukemia, sleep apnea, or whatever, was fixed. This is not a rare occurrence.

One thing's for sure. When someone finally evaluates cases like this and finds a serious cause for what they thought to be migraine ordinaire, it wasn't a duck that suffered the consequences. It was a person who had a disease that someone missed, and may have needed treatment long ago. Unfortunate cases like this are trying to tell us that there's some kind of faulty reasoning in our approach. How could that be?

Here's one way it might happen: Imagine a person walks in the door with a headache that fits the definition of migraine perfectly. You use the walks-like-a-duck reasoning and conclude, "It's migraine. The rule is: we don't do a scan for migraine." Your reasoning goes like this: "You fit the definition perfectly, so you have migraine. Migraine is what we call a primary headache, which means that you have an innate susceptibility to this kind of headache and that there is no serious underlying cause. So we don't do a scan. We treat the headache. I'll give you a prescription for Topamax, the treatment of choice."

This is a textbook example of circular reasoning. You start out by saying that the thing you need to prove is true, which leads to the conclusion that you don't have to prove it. "Why work it up if we're not going to do anything about it anyway." has this same kind of erroneous reasoning embedded in it. I'm left thinking, "You're amazing. You have the uncanny ability to know that we don't have to treat something, even when you don't know what it is that we don't have to treat!" This kind of thinking is common in medicine today.

> **"You're amazing. You have an uncanny ability to know that we don't have to treat something, even when you don't know what it is that we don't have to treat!"**

True, there are reasons we might not evaluate a headache that fits the definition of migraine. When we do this, we must keep in mind that we have not done the workup to prove it. So I call headaches like this migraine-like, migrainous headache or *presumed* migraine, not migraine. You've seen how important it is to know underlying cause or at least say that you don't know the cause when it wasn't evaluated. A lot hangs on this idea of knowing the underlying cause.

Primary and secondary headache: The idea that a headache can be just a symptom of some underlying cause is not new. It's embodied in the concept of idiopathic and symptomatic headaches proposed by Christian Baur in 1787. Idiopathic means that the disease you are speaking of has no known cause. Symptomatic, as the term is used here, means that the headache is a symptom of an underlying disorder. My understanding of Baur's thinking goes like this: If you can identify a tumor, an infection or some tangible cause for the headache, then it's a symptomatic headache. The headache caused by a tumor is called a symptomatic headache because it is a symptom of the tumor. If you cannot identify a cause for the headache, well, that's what idiopathic means, so you call it an idiopathic headache. This means "I don't know what the cause of this headache is." Using Baur's definition, migraine and tension-type headaches are called idiopathic headaches.

I don't like the word idiopathic because it's often thought of as a diagnosis. If we write "idiopathic headache" in the chart, say, "Come back in three months." and go on to the next patient, we've ended the search for a diagnosis.

I prefer to write "Headache of unknown cause." That's even better than calling it migrainous headache because *unknown* is a word making it clear that "We're not finished yet. We're still trying to find the cause."

Baur's concept has evolved into a more useful one, which we use today: the notion of primary and secondary headaches.

A primary headache is an innate characteristic of the person. Migraine, tension-type headache and cluster headache are primary headaches. A person is born with a susceptibility to these headaches; they're part of their makeup. They may be triggered by certain foods, stress, maybe other things, but there's no underlying process or disorder that we can ever find and fix. So we wind up treating the headache.

A secondary headache is caused by some underlying disorder, usually something that's acquired after we are born. So headaches caused by a brain tumor, high pressure inside the head, trauma and infection are examples of secondary headaches. When evaluation reveals the underlying cause, our treatment is mainly directed to the cause, not the headache. The headache is just a symptom of the underlying cause.

All headaches are secondary: As I see it, all headaches are secondary, even those we call primary headaches. This became clear to me in the success stories. Most of the cases were migraineurs who had little benefit from eliminating triggers or using the preventative medications. They didn't get better until I found and corrected the underlying cause. Then the improvement was dramatic.

Not only that, but also the strong response to treatment defined the pathogenesis. When sleep improved and migraine

> **I don't like the word idiopathic because it's often thought of as a diagnosis. I prefer to write "Headache of unknown cause." Unknown is a word making it clear that "We're not finished yet.**

resolved on Depakote or lithium or Lamictal and the patient returned saying, "When I sleep, I don't get headaches," I could be reasonably certain that a subtle form of the manic trait was the underlying cause. I also knew exactly how it caused the headaches. We have already seen in *Vivacious* how mania activated migraine, and in others how worry activated migraine. Here we see temporal lobe epilepsy activating something that looks just like migraine. This means that even the primary headaches have underlying mechanisms that can be defined. Treatment directed to the cause was more effective than treatment directed at the headache. That's because the headache is only a symptom of its underlying cause.

So Baur's concept and even today's concept of primary and secondary headaches has done us a disservice. When it's a primary headache, these concepts turn our attention to treating the headache, and end the search for an underlying cause. Most headaches are called primary headaches today, so this disservice applies to most of those we treat.

A headache is only a symptom of its underlying cause.

Thinking "pathogenesis": This is an important case because it shows that not only does migraine masquerade as other things, the opposite is also true. In this case, temporal lobe epilepsy took on the appearance of migraine. Many other things may look like migraine. We can make a mistake both ways.

It also gave occasion to rethink the concepts of primary and secondary headaches and how easy it is to slip into a mindset that doesn't look any farther when we conclude that our patient has one of the primary headaches. What primary headache means to me now is that the person has an inherited, innate susceptibility to his or her particular kind of headache. If it's a susceptibility to migraine, that migraine process can be activated by many things, all the way from triggers like heat and sun and alcohol to more important things like depletion and emotions and even to critical things like epilepsy. The susceptibility to migraine varies from person to person. It may even change through a lifetime.

It also shows that the best way to uncover the pathogenesis of a headache is to assume from the start that all headaches are secondary. This important assumption encourages us to begin with the search for pathogenesis.

Here's something interesting: Notice that I never had to treat this young fellow's headaches. They stopped when we treated the epilepsy.

Idiopathic Intracranial Hypertension (IIH)

Migraine is common, but we can't just go around calling everything migraine. Mixed in with the common headaches are a few that are serious. We've just seen how epilepsy can cause headaches that look just like migraine. It also happens that headaches are called migraine when they obviously are something else.

We can't call everything migraine. Mixed in with the common headaches are a few that are serious.

Swooshing: A young woman with headache "all over my head" and episodes in which "The vision in my right eye goes dark." was seen in two emergency departments and diagnosed with migraine each time. They treated her as such, although she told them that she didn't think it was migraine. She'd never had migraine before and she didn't have the typical sensitivity to light and nausea so characteristic of migraine. The headaches started three months earlier, never went away and were steadily getting worse. She was a little overweight. Well, more than a little. Understandably, she was worried.

My first question: "Do you ever hear a swooshing sound in your head?"

"How did you know that? At first, I'd hear it in bed when the house was quiet. Now I have it all the time. It's driving me crazy. How do I get rid of it?"

She was describing a *bruit* (pronounced bru-ee), a swooshing sound, in-time with her heartbeat. The patient can hear this kind of bruit. The doctor cannot. I've had it once in a while with a bad migraine, but most of the time when a person describes a bruit it means he or she has high pressure in his or her head for some reason. It's more prominent when a person is flat in bed because the pressure inside the head normally increases when you're flat and decreases when you stand up. A bruit like this is a marker for elevated intracranial pressure, which is usually caused by what's called idiopathic intracranial hypertension (IIH). Other names for the same thing are pseudotumor cerebri and benign intracranial hypertension. This is something different from what is usually called hypertension, meaning high arterial blood pressure. IIH means that there is high spinal fluid pressure in the head.

A few days after the ED visits she saw an optometrist because her eye began to go dark many times a day. He found swollen optic discs and gave me a call. I saw her a few hours later.

When I see an overweight woman of childbearing age with a new headache, the first thing that comes to mind is IIH. The first question I ask is, "Do you ever hear a swooshing sound in your head?"

Then the next thing I do is pick up an ophthalmoscope and examine the inside of her eyes. The optometrist was right, both optic nerves were swollen. She had papilledema, which means swollen optic nerves, a sign of high pressure inside the head. "Did anyone in emergency look into your eyes?" She didn't think so. Papilledema is easily missed in the emergency room.

IIH can have serious consequences. When papilledema gets bad enough and persists long enough, it causes permanent damage to the optic nerves, which means permanent loss of vision, in a young person no less.

Her MRI was normal except for prominent spinal fluid rings around each optic nerve and what's called an empty sella, signs that confirm longstanding high intracranial pressure. There was no tumor. A spinal tap showed that the pressure in her head was about as high as one can measure. Spinal fluid analysis was normal; so the diagnosis of IIH was made.

Years ago we called IIH pseudotumor cerebri. Pseudo indicates that the high pressure is not caused by a tumor. Before we had CT and MRI scans, there was often a lingering question of tumor. So we used the word pseudotumor to make it clear what we thought we were treating.

There is debate over what causes IIH. The "idiopathic" part of IIH means that the cause is not known. We typically see it in overweight women of childbearing age, especially when they gain weight and over-hydrate or become pregnant. My theory is this: In most cases, IIH happens when a person is born with unusually small veins that drain blood from the brain. The pressure inside a person's head is roughly equal to venous pressure. So anything that increases venous pressure inside the head will also increase intracranial spinal fluid pressure. We can demonstrate this during a spinal tap with the Queckenstedt maneuver.

As my theory of IIH goes, a person with IIH is born with somewhat high intracranial pressure because venous outflow from the brain is insufficient. Then, if the pressure inside the chest (where venous blood goes) increases by gaining weight, becoming pregnant or over-hydrating, the pressure inside their head goes even higher. Only then does the pressure get high enough to cause papilledema, headaches and a bruit.

It was no surprise when my patient commented, "I drink loads of water." as she reached for the bottle of water that she was working on. The usual treatment for IIH is Diamox and dehydration by restricting salt and fluid until weight loss brings the person to a normal body mass index. As I say, all this is controversial. I found some weak support for my theory when the husband of one of my IIH patients commented as they walked out the door, "Honey, it's the pizza."

Red flags

What can we learn here? No doubt about it, this story is all about recognizing the red flags of a serious headache and, when your doctors don't recognize them, trusting in yourself enough to seek further evaluation.

The history is loaded with red flags for serious headache. First, this was a new headache in someone who said, "I don't get headaches." Second, the headache did not have any earmarks of migraine, her emergency department diagnoses. They were not episodic or one-sided, no nausea or sensitivity to light. No one asked if she heard a bruit and apparently no one did an eye exam to spot the papilledema. Maybe they did the eye exam. If they did, they must have missed the papilledema. Surely it was present if she was having episodes of loss of vision. All this in a person who is a dead-ringer for IIH: obese female of child-bearing age with a new headache who even tells you, "It isn't migraine." Her opinion must have been worth something.

The transient visual blackouts are a sign that the swollen optic nerve is losing blood supply because the pressure is so high. This led to evaluation by the optometrist who saw the papilledema and made the urgent referral.

Aside from the necessity of looking into the eye to rule out papilledema in anyone who has headache, this case shows how important it is to look for red flags, trouble signs of a more serious process causing the headache. She had many red flags.

In addition to the bruit, new headache and loss of vision, other red flags of raised intracranial pressure may be present. These include muffled hearing caused by stretching of the eighth

This story is about recognizing the red flags of a serious headache. When your doctors don't recognize them, trust in yourself enough to seek further evaluation.

cranial nerve, double vision caused by sixth cranial nerve palsies and even bradycardia, a slow heart rate, when the tenth cranial nerve is stretched by the high intracranial pressure. Loss of vision is the critical red flag, however, because it indicates imminent loss of vision that may be permanent.

Facial Pain, HSV and Trigeminal Neuralgia

Here's another entity that's often overlooked or misdiagnosed. A quick pickup and treatment can save the patient considerable anguish.

Psychotherapist: I walked into the room, looked at her chart and saw that she was a psychotherapist. Being an electrical engineer who didn't do particularly well in the social skills department, I have to admit that I'm a little intimidated by psychotherapists. The first thing I said, with a bit of hesitation in my voice, "Now, before we begin . . . just to get the record straight . . . one thing you need to know . . . I'm an . . . electrical engineer." Relieved, I said to myself, "There, I said it."

With a confident smile and a knowing look, she replied, "Oh. I won't expect social skills then." Suddenly I felt at ease. She understood me. I never cease to be amazed at how good psychotherapists are at things like that.

Two years earlier she had developed pain in the left side of her face extending down into her neck and left arm. Thinking that a slipped disc was the cause, she had a cervical fusion without much benefit. When the pain persisted and extended into her tongue as a numb, tingling sensation, she saw a neurosurgeon who diagnosed "atypical facial pain" and began Trileptal as symptomatic treatment.

I saw her for the first time one year later. The pain had become severe and was now focused in her left eye.

First question: "Do you get cold sores?"

"Yes. I have them often. In fact, I had one just a few months ago. Why do you ask?"

"Most likely, the cause of your pain is herpes simplex virus, HSV for short."

A cold sore is a painful sore on the edge of the lip or nose caused by the herpes simplex virus, also known as HSV. (In contrast, sores that occur inside the mouth are usually canker sores, something different.) Herpes simplex virus lives in the trigeminal nerve, the fifth cranial nerve, which carries touch and pain sensation from everything in the front of the head: face, mouth, and deeper structures including the front of the brain and the remainder of the cranial nerves two through twelve. So the virus has a connection to many structures: the eye, blood vessels, other cranial nerves, you name it. Brain tissue itself doesn't have trigeminal innervation. When the virus replicates (reproduces) it may cause a tingling, painful sore on the margin of your lip if it reaches the surface of the skin. When the virus becomes active deep in the nerve, painful inflammation occurs without a visible cold sore. HSV is a frequent cause of eye pain, loss of vision and loss of function in other cranial nerves.

Often overlooked

HSV infections are common, the most common cause of trigeminal neuralgia in my experience. I think it was the usual cause of what we called "atypical facial pain" years ago. We just never knew it because there's no easy way to be sure it's HSV. When herpes erupts on the skin, we can take a small sample and do cultures or antibody and DNA tests to be sure. Most of the time, however, there's no rash or cold sore. So how do we know it's HSV?

Even though it isn't easy to prove that HSV is the cause of the problem, four things make HSV the prime suspect:

1) There is often a history of cold sores. If the person has had many cold sores over years, HSV is highly suspect.

2) If the virus is actively replicating, the pain and neurological symptoms show a dramatic response to Valtrex, an antiviral for herpes viruses, in about 36 hours.

3) Herpes simplex antibodies in the blood indicate that a person has was exposed to HSV. The immune system is responding. If the antibody titer is high, the immune system is responding strongly, a sign of recent viral activity. Antiviral treatment with Valtrex stops viral replication, but does not kill the virus. The herpesvirus remains dormant until it is activated again for some reason. Scans and bloodwork are usually normal otherwise.

4) If HSV is causing nerve pain, what we call neuralgia, the pain almost always responds to an adequate dose of gabapentin[4]. If it doesn't respond to gabapentin dramatically, the dose was too

Herpesvirus infections are the most common cause of trigeminal neuralgia in my experience, and they are easily treated. Unfortunately, they often go unrecognized.

4. **Gabapentin** is a relatively safe and highly effective treatment for neuropathic pain, pain caused by a disorder of body (somatic) sensation. It is especially effective for the pain of herpesvirus infections. It is excreted through the kidneys so it's effect is short, about 6 hours. It probably reduces pain by binding to the $\alpha 2\delta$ receptor in the dorsal horn of the spinal cord where pain sensation is processed.

low or the pain is not herpesvirus neuralgia.

Easily treated

I've included this case because herpesvirus infections are common and easily treated. Unfortunately, they often go unrecognized for years, two years in this case. During this time, the herpesvirus may recur in waves, called relapses, two or three times a year. In the meantime, permanent injury can occur to the nerve and the eye leaving a person in a chronic state of pain called post-herpetic neuralgia, with loss of vision or a multitude of other problems. This is a potentially serious headache.

If there's a high index of suspicion for herpesvirus, I begin Valtrex immediately and then do the testing. A good response to Valtrex has diagnostic value and gives the best chance of avoiding serious and permanent neurological problems. I also do a gabapentin trial. One of our most effective medications for the pain of neuralgia, gabapentin is one of the safest medications I know. It doesn't help migraine, muscle pain, sinus pain or the headache of high intracranial pressure very much, so a good response to gabapentin means that the pain is most likely neuralgia. The trial has diagnostic value. Exactly how gabapentin and Valtrex are used is important, but beyond the scope of this book.

I asked my patient the psychotherapist to begin both Valtrex and gabapentin immediately and sent blood for antibodies to HSV.

Dramatic response: She was lucky. Her pain responded to gabapentin and resolved completely on Valtrex. She didn't need more than a dose or two of gabapentin, but I continued Valtrex for a while so that recurrent HSV activity would not interfere with her recovery. HSV titers were high as expected. The high titers, history of cold sores and the good response to gabapentin and Valtrex provide good presumptive evidence that HSV was indeed the cause of all her symptoms, including the left arm pain. Explaining this is also beyond the scope of this book. Let me just say that herpesviruses can affect nerves anywhere in the body.

She left with an interesting comment, "I've seen so many doctors for this. No one put me on Valtrex." I guess it took an engineer.

I asked her to keep a few Valtrex on hand. At the first sign of any HSV recurrence, take a few doses. Usually that's all you need.

A price to pay: Herpesvirus infections are common and underrecognized. There is often a delay in beginning treatment and the consequences can be serious, including chronic pain called post herpetic neuralgia and loss of vision. To complicate matters, there are many kinds of herpesvirus. They present in strange ways, so it's hard to know for sure that a herpesvirus is causing the problem. The patients bounce around from doctor to doctor until; finally, someone stumbles onto the answer.

Red Eye: A 26-year-old young man came from far away for a painful, red eye that just wasn't getting better. He had been in and out of emergency departments and the hospital, and treated with several antibiotics and steroids to no avail. By the time we saw him, morphine could no longer control the pain. The best word I can think of to describe the eye is scary. The white of the eye was blood red and swollen. He was so sensitive to light that I couldn't even check his pupils. His face was numb to touch around the eye. Ah! A clue: the trigeminal nerve is involved.

I was ahead of the game when he arrived because I already knew that he didn't respond to potent antibiotics or steroids. So it was probably not a bacterial infection, Tolosa Hunt or an autoimmune process of some kind.

My first question, "Do you get cold sores?"

"A lot." The history was just a few words here and there in answer to my questions. He was in that much pain.

I asked my clinical assistant, "What's your best guess?" He's pre-med, which means that he's a medical school hopeful. He hasn't been there yet.

"Just one thing, Dr. Smith: HSV." His exact words; my thinking exactly. In just six months, my pre-med clinical assistant had seen so many variations of HSV that he could spot it at a glance.

On Valtrex, the red eye cleared within a few days, leaving him with severe post-herpetic neuralgia. Although the eye was quiet, I wasn't able to manage his pain, so I sent him to the hospital. After a 10 day admission, I got a call from a rather distinguished, senior hospitalist, "What a fascinating case! Never in my whole career have I seen anything like this." I thought, "My clinical assistant diagnosed him at the snap of a finger."

Do you see what I mean when I say "under-recognized?" In part, that's because there is an wide spectrum of disorders caused by herpesviruses. It goes well beyond anything you find in the textbooks. Furthermore, it isn't possible to prove that a herpesvirus was the cause in most cases. This uncertainty diminishes our ability to identify the cause.

Three types of herpesvirus account for most of the herpes infections we see: 1) herpes simplex-1 (HSV-1) the cold sore virus, 2) herpes simplex-2 (HSV-2) the genital herpesvirus and 3) varicella zoster virus (VZV) the chickenpox/shingles virus. Pain, often severe, is common to all. Bloodwork and scans often do not show an abnormality except for elevated antibody titers to the virus. I have found that any cranial nerve can be affected except cranial nerve 1. There is often no rash. The best confirmation, if you can't get a culture or DNA test, is high serum IgG antibody titers and a good response to Valtrex. Pain may persist after treatment if there are delays in starting an antiviral.

An Abnormal Finding

"It's easier to diagnose and treat the headache of a brain tumor than a migraine." I can't count the number of times I've made that comment. In medicine, we use the term "lesion" to say we found an abnormal area on exam or a scan. The word suggests that we don't know what it is. So, when we say that the MRI scan shows a lesion, it means that the scan shows a "something." It might be a tumor, an aneurysm, an area of inflammation. A lesion is a structural problem; it's concrete. Something is there, and we feel reassured that "I found something." (Often we say "lesion" in a general way even when we know what it is, in much the same way that I might say "headache" when I'm discussing migraine.)

Even when there's a lesion on the MRI scan, it isn't always clear whether it's causing the headaches.

Out on a limb

Even when there's a lesion on the MRI scan, it isn't always clear whether it's causing the headaches. It could just be an incidental finding that has nothing to do with them. Consider this for example.

Charleston: In my younger years, ballroom dancing

was what I did for fun. I took lessons in foxtrot, waltz and quickstep from a woman who was in her 70s. One day she appeared in my office with low back pain, so severe that she couldn't teach. I sent her for an MRI scan that day. Looking at the films I commented, "Lena, you've got the worst spinal stenosis I've ever seen. It's no wonder you're having so much back pain. You need surgery."

"David, I'm too old for surgery. What else can I do?"

I thought for a minute. "Well, maybe your pain has an arthritic component. A single dose of prednisone will take that away for a day or two, and then at least you know how much of the pain is coming from arthritis and how much is coming from the spinal stenosis."

I wrote a script for prednisone, and she returned in a week to say that the prednisone didn't change a thing.

"Lena, you need surgery."

"I told you. I'm too old for surgery. What else can I do?"

I was a little frustrated. "Well . . . Why don't you go home and get into a tub of hot water? When your back muscles are nice and warm, do stretching exercises in the tub. If you feel a little better after that, then some of the pain is muscular . . . but Lena, you need surgery."

She didn't come back after that. Two months later I went to a dance, and there was Lena and her partner in the middle of the floor demonstrating the Charleston, and a fast one at that.

When she finished, I sauntered over with a nervous smile. "How's your back?"

"I went home that day and got right into a tub of hot water and did the range of motion you suggested. I felt a little better when I got out. I'm retired now, so I could do the tub therapy four or five times a day. After a few of weeks the pain was gone!"

When Lena was on the dance floor doing the Charleston, she had the same spinal stenosis that she had when she came in with so much pain. So the spinal stenosis wasn't the cause of her pain after all. It was muscular. Lena is 90 now. She never had back surgery and still doesn't need it.

I would have sent her for failed surgery had she not insisted otherwise. It was a sobering lesson that's made me ask time and again, ". . . but is that lesion we see on the scan really causing the symptoms?" It's a good question to keep in mind regardless of whether it's a likely or unlikely cause of symptoms.

Persistence pays off

Arachnoid Cyst: A six-year-old boy came with Mom and Dad for evaluation of developmental delays. He was born a twin by C-section, had good APGARs and developed normally until age two when he began to stutter. In kindergarten, he seemed to have fine motor and perceptual delays confirmed on formal testing, although he demonstrated high intelligence otherwise. His biggest complaint was frequent headaches.

MRI of the head was normal except for a 2.3 cm water-filled cyst near his mesial temporal lobe, a part of the brain that mediates emotions and memory and is especially susceptible to epilepsy. We discussed the remote possibility that the arachnoid cyst was causing his symptoms and agreed on a repeat MRI in two years to see if the cyst was expanding. "Return sooner if the headaches get worse."

I next saw him 4 years later. Now ten he was diagnosed with generalized anxiety disorder and depression and the fine motor and perceptual deficits had become more prominent. He had two or three headaches a month easily terminated with medication. He occasionally had episodes of unprovoked rage. I asked if he smelled things that weren't there. He said, "Yes." He couldn't identify the smell, but it was definitely not pleasant.

Repeat MRI showed no change in the cyst. EEG was normal, no evidence for a seizure disorder.

We saw in the case of *Special Ed* that a weird smell, an uncinate aura, is a tip-off for temporal lobe epilepsy. Unprovoked rage is another. Perhaps the EEG missed it.

I started a low dose of Tegretol, an antiepileptic drug (AED) that makes just about anyone more resistant to seizures. His headaches stopped, mood improved, schoolwork improved and there were no more episodes of rage or unpleasant smells.

During the next two years, he had repeat EEG's, neurosurgical consults, five-day EEG monitoring, pediatric-neuro consults and out of town evaluations in Baltimore and Pittsburgh. Everyone who saw him found "No evidence to support a diagnosis of epilepsy." There I was, unable to get him off anticonvulsants. Every time I tried, the headaches returned, mood and cognitive function deteriorated and the uncinate auras returned, an example of the cross-correlation technique mentioned in Chapter 2. So I sent him to Cleveland Clinic for what was by then a tenth opinion.

He was admitted. The next day the neurologist in Cleveland called, "Could I insert a sphenoid electrode?" This is a wire that passes under the skull-base to record from the mesial temporal lobe, the location of the cyst. That's also the area of the brain that generates the uncinate aura and the rage.

"Of course."

A few hours later Cleveland called back to say that the sphenoid electrode had recorded epileptic discharges originating in the left temporal lobe, clear evidence of temporal lobe seizure activity at the site of the arachnoid cyst! So now we knew why the anticonvulsants worked so well.

Over the next eight months, he required increasing doses of AEDs. The cyst was completely removed with a minimally invasive technique. At last report, he was doing quite well in school, mood was normal and uncinate auras and headaches were long-gone, on half the dose of AED he required pre-op.

Temporal lobe seizures are common in a neurology practice, usually have a psychiatric look and are easy to miss on EEG. That's because the mesial temporal lobe is deep within the head and surface electrodes cannot pick up electrical activity there unless the seizure activity spreads to areas near the scalp electrodes. So temporal lobe seizures can be hard to diagnose. More than once, I've seen them ruin a young person's 12 years of education.

You would be amazed at the list of this young fellow's misdiagnoses, including a psychiatric diagnosis or two. They were examples of *unreasonable certainty*. The EEG in Cleveland proved them all wrong. It would have been better to replace all these misdiagnoses with the diagnosis "cause unknown." At least that would have kept his doctors looking.

You've seen in some of the earlier stories how the emotional or what we call psychosocial part of an illness is under-recognized. In this case, I'm saying the opposite: the emotional part was over-diagnosed. The emotional problems in this case were part of a biological, not a psychological, problem. This biological problem was temporal lobe epilepsy caused by the pressure of an arachnoid cyst on the mesial temporal lobe. When the pressure was removed surgically, the emotions returned to normal.

> **It would have been better to replace all the misdiagnoses with the words "cause unknown."**

A different kind of payoff

What I'm saying is that, paradoxically, the emotional part of an illness is both under-recognized and over-diagnosed. If we agree with this, we must resist the temptation to be certain about the diagnosis when certainty is not there. Instead of closing the case by saying "it's this" or "it's that," at times it's best to say "I just don't know." This kind of uncertainty makes some people very uncomfortable, doctor and patient alike.

> **Paradoxically, the emotional part of an illness is both under-recognized and over-diagnosed.**

> *Asymmetric Ventricles:* A 43-year-old woman came for migraine, migraine from hell. In her teens, she had sensitivity to light, nausea, tunnel vision and even episodes of loss of consciousness. All that went away for about 20 years. One month before I first saw her, it all returned. In fact, she had four episodes of loss of consciousness during the prior month.
>
> She was hit by a truck 12 years earlier and paralyzed from the waist down for six weeks. No headache with that. Sleep has never been good. She had a number of other medical problems including a pulmonary embolism. She had a clean lifestyle and a devoted husband. She was idealistic, very intelligent and gave a lot back to her community. She took a big bite out of life. There was considerable stress.
>
> A mega-workup was negative, although when we reviewed her MRI scans, I noticed that the right ventricle was larger than the left. I made the comment, "Not a likely cause of any headaches. I'm sure this is some form of

migraine, probably basilar artery migraine in view of your tunnel vision and the episodes of loss of consciousness."

I took a biopsychosocial approach, looking for ways to reduce stress, and even saw her with her husband. We did several medication trials for migraine, worry, sleep disorder, raised intracranial pressure and even manic illness. I tried every trick in the book, left no stone unturned. Nothing helped. Every week or two she either popped into the office in severe, severe migraine status that could be terminated only with double doses of Dilaudid and Phenergan or went to emergency for the same thing.

I began to wonder if this were migraine. I was certain that she was not drug-seeking. Could she intermittently be obstructing her large right ventricle? Her headaches went from zero to severe very quickly, a characteristic of ventricular obstruction called *square headache*.

I sent her to a neurosurgeon for a second opinion, the best I know for ventricular problems. He was sure that the ventricular asymmetry was not causing headaches, no surgery needed. I was stuck.

After six months of this, I didn't hear from my patient for a few months; very odd. I was about to call to find what's going on, when one day there she was, sitting in the exam room.

"My headaches are gone." was the first thing she said, now with a peaceful countenance.

"What happened?"

She had an epiphany, a realization that her life was just too much. Too many committees with too much committee work, too much stress at home, too much stress everywhere. She resigned from the boards she had been on and declined an offer for admission to a PhD program with full scholarship. She kept her family.

There she was, headache-free for more than a month; another triumph for the Wright brothers' principle! What's more, she came up with the answer on her own. It wasn't her ventricles after all.

You can see that this business of diagnosis can be a treacherous landscape to navigate. More than just pain, headaches can become so incapacitating that a person cannot even go to school or function as a mom or dad. That creates a crisis. A lot of testing gets done.

If there's still no answer, doctor and patient get desperate. If the patient isn't getting better, procedures and surgery might be done, medication might be given that may have serious consequences.

Having been through a number of these situations, I can say this: Just because we find something wrong doesn't mean that it's causing the problem. When emotions are involved, doctors are quick to call it psychiatric. Second opinions are valuable, but they are only opinions. They aren't always correct.

Just because we find something wrong doesn't mean that it's causing the problem.

Fortunately, serious headaches are not common. Even so, most would agree that simply saying a serious cause is unlikely is not good reason to forego evaluation.

Chapter Five

Baffling Headaches

The headaches that nobody can figure out, they're the ones that really teach us something

A good feeling always accompanies a solved headache case. The feeling I get when I finally discover the cause of a headache that's baffled me for a while . . . well, that's pure elation.

Basilar Artery Migraine Equivalent

We began Chapter 3 with a case of masquerade migraine. Here we see how good the disguise can be.

> *Seven Years of Hell:* "I was perfectly healthy until November 2002. All of a sudden one night I woke up with an attack of wild spinning and vomiting. The sound in my right ear was muffled, and for a day or two I couldn't even walk; I was that dizzy. It was two weeks before I could function again. Since then, it's been seven years of hell."
>
> She was a pleasant, clean-living 54-year-old woman who came with a concerned husband. She was having recurrent episodes of severe vertigo since the onset, now with persistent and progressive hearing loss in the right ear. She had seen two of the best ENT specialists and a neurologist, been evaluated for Ménière's disease and multiple sclerosis, had vestibular therapy and been on a variety of medications to the point of being "a walking zombie." Nothing helped. She was about to have a cochlear implant for the hearing loss.
>
> My first thought: "Sounds like basilar artery migraine." I looked at her husband. "Do you have any insight into what might be going on?"

"Whatever it is, this is some kind of process that's been going on most of her life. This isn't something that started in 2002. In her 30s she had mild attacks of vertigo that kept happening up till the bad one in 2002."

She agreed and added that since childhood she's always been carsick and couldn't even look at whirling rides in the amusement park, let alone go on them; just about anything seemed to trigger these episodes of vertigo. "Could it be menopause?" she asked.

Both agreed that she was a worrier, conscientious, a caregiver and had very strong emotional responses to things. Today's office visit was stressful enough to cause her face and neck to turn bright red. Her husband took a look and said, "That's how she is."

In the first five minutes of the history I'm thinking, "This doesn't sound like any Ménière's disease that I've ever seen. The symptoms have sudden onset, then gradually fade. That's a vascular tempo, the way a stroke behaves. If she's had these episodes for 20 years, it's not likely that she's about to have a stroke. She wasn't menopausal in her amusement park days. It sounds like vasospasm more than anything else I know. The symptoms are brainstem symptoms, so it's sounding more like basilar artery migraine by the minute. She had markers for migraine, dizziness at the amusement park and often carsick, when she was little. She's also an emotionally responsive individual. The facial flushing tells me that a strong autonomic response comes along with the emotions. It sure sounds like Bickerstaff's basilar artery migraine. Some of his cases had persistent brainstem symptoms just like this. Migraine would also explain why her husband thought that this was a lifelong process."

"Do you get headaches?"
"No. No headaches at all."

So these probably are basilar artery migraine without the headache, what we might call basilar artery migraine equivalents.

"Have you ever been on verapamil?"
"Never."

Verapamil blocks vasospasm. If my hypothesis is correct, it should fix the problem. Two weeks later, on a low dose of verapamil, she returned.

"I can't believe this! Only one episode; and that was after I missed a dose. I'm feeling so much better."

She also said on this visit that the verapamil fixed her irritable bowel, a marker for vasospasm. I presume the vasospasm is caused by a calcium channelopathy, an inborn anomaly of calcium channels that makes the muscles in arteries that cause vasospasm unusually irritable.

"You've probably inherited three things: First, a susceptibility to the migraine mechanism which, in you, happens without headache. Second, a calcium channelopathy that makes you susceptible to vasospasm and often accompanies the migraine. It's a form of migraine called basilar artery migraine. It also causes Prinzmetal's angina, when there's vasospasm in the coronary arteries, and even irritable bowel. Finally, you inherited an emotionally responsive personality with a tendency to worry. Strong emotions cause adrenaline surges that trigger the vasospasm. I even wonder if the vertigo that wakes you at night is caused by strong adrenaline surges when you sleep, much the same as a person who wakes with panic attacks. We often see bursts of rapid heart rate on overnight pulse oximetry caused by these adrenaline surges."

I hope it doesn't sound immodest to say that her dramatic change for the better was no accident. The striking thing about this case isn't that she was cured; it's how quickly that happened. How can a person have immediate recognition of the underlying cause when her diagnosis had stumped a number of very capable physicians for years? Again that word pops into my head, "Why?"

I'm still trying to understand what happened here, but I have an idea about the "Why." of it. One thing that's different about me; I just can't say "I don't know . . . Come back in three months." I'm compelled to keep searching until I understand. I can't let an unsolved mystery go. It's like the *Sip of Coffee* story, that day when I was out in the garage. Except there's a difference: Every time I finish my diagnostic sip of coffee, I mean every time I figure something out, I learn something that helps with the next case. This gracious woman was a good example. I was quickly able to recognize the pathogenesis in her case because I had figured out

The striking thing about this case isn't that she was cured; it's how quickly that happened. Every time I figure something out, I learn something that helps with the next case.

variations of this theme many times before. I puzzled for a while the first time I saw something like this, but then with each case the diagnosis came easier and easier. After years of this, a person comes to learn some things that aren't in the textbooks.

Hypoxia Headache

Lack of oxygen, hypoxia for short, occurs in different ways. None of them are good for you. Several things happen after years of smoking that come together, like the perfect storm, to create a critical lack of oxygen and with it, headaches.

> *Yosemite Sam:* Some years ago I saw a testy fellow in his 40s with "God-awful headaches." Again, no one could fix them. When I say testy, I mean it. He was a scary kind of fellow. Early on, he let me know, "I'll kill anybody who gets in my way!" He made it clear that I might be next if I couldn't fix his headaches. The first image that comes to mind for this fellow is the Looney Tunes character Yosemite Sam. He even looked a little like him.
>
> I wasn't sure exactly what kind of headache he had. It was severe, all over his head, got better and worse but never went away and wasn't associated with the usual migraine markers, sensitivity to light and nausea. It had steadily grown worse over a year or so. In fact, it was so bad that he hadn't been able to work for the year before I saw him.
>
> He had a smoker's face and smelled like a cigarette, so it wasn't hard to guess that he was a heavy smoker. "I smoke two, maybe three, sometimes more, packs a day." Whatever that meant, it sure looked like he smoked a lot.

The first thing I do when someone smokes is get a serum carboxyhemoglobin and order overnight pulse oximetry. Carboxyhemoglobin is a measure of carbon monoxide in the blood, which occurs with smoking. Overnight pulse oximetry measures how much oxygen is in the blood while a person is sleeping. Blood oxygen levels are their best when a person is awake. Blood oxygen saturation, or SpO_2, drops during sleep because respiratory drive normally decreases during sleep. Years of smoking also change the upper airway to cause snoring and obstructive sleep apnea. The lung damage further decreases SpO_2.

In this case, the pulse oximetry showed a low baseline oxygen saturation (SpO2) = 89%. In a healthy young person it usually runs about 94% during sleep. Anything below 88% raises concern. So his SpO2 was marginal at best, indicating that he had early emphysema from years of smoking. On top of that, he had episodes of severe obstructive sleep apnea that briefly brought his SpO2 down much lower.

There was yet another problem. His blood carboxyhemoglobin showed that more than 15% of the hemoglobin in his red blood cells was tied up in carbon monoxide. Most pulse oximeters read carbon monoxide as oxygen, so his true SpO2 was about 15% less or 74%. That was his baseline! When he obstructed, his true oxygen saturation dropped below 60%. Altogether, this means that he was sleeping with blood oxygen at times equivalent to an altitude of 18,000 feet!

If no one can figure out the cause of your headaches and you smoke heavily You might have your answer right there.

Oxygen levels this low can cause permanent loss of vision and even brain damage. To understand how this relates to his headaches, I have to tell you a story of my own.

> *Altitude Headache:* I belong to the North American Neuro-Ophthalmology Society, NANOS for short. They often hold their meetings in ski country because most of the members like to ski. I don't ski. In my ballroom dancing days, I promised myself never to ski because if I injured my knee, I wouldn't be able to foxtrot any more.
>
> So what I do at NANOS meetings is go around all week with an altitude headache, up there at 9000 feet. The point I'm trying to make is that lack of oxygen gives many people a headache. Whether you call this migraine or altitude headache or something else isn't that important. What's important is that Yosemite Sam was in effect sleeping above 18,000 feet at times during the night. His hypoxia was severe enough to cause neurological damage, let alone give him a headache. The Federal Aviation Administration requires a pilot to use oxygen above 12,500 feet.

I fixed my altitude headaches by taking Diamox. It's a diuretic that makes the body slightly more acidic. Called *metabolic acidosis*, I presume this makes a person over-breathe a little and thereby raises the blood oxygen enough to prevent altitude headaches. I do tingle a bit from the Diamox and carbonated beverages don't taste right, but that's a small price to pay for no headache.

Diamox wouldn't be enough to help my patient, so I gave him nasal oxygen at night at a high flow rate. After a week of that he returned with his headaches more than 50% better, although I had to pull it out of him. I don't think he wanted to admit that I found the principal cause of his headaches because it meant that he needed to quit smoking.

If no one can figure out the cause of your headaches and you smoke heavily, get a serum carboxyhemoglobin and overnight pulse oximetry. You might have your answer right there.

Closing Doors

I'm not sure if the word "no" causes headaches, but I do know that this word can be a baffling reason why they don't get better. Here's how it happens.

"No." in the Air: In my early days of practice, I saw a woman in her 30s who came from afar, hoping to find someone who could cure her headaches. She seemed well put together, in control and was a highly intelligent person. She held a responsible position that capitalized on that intelligence.

There wasn't much question that she had migraine. The headaches started in her teens. Over recent years they had become more severe and frequent often interfering with her ability to work, although she never missed work. She had the usual bloodwork and scans, which were all negative and had tried a few medications and seen many doctors, but never with any success.

At the end of the visit, I suggested that instead of searching for a treatment, we try to find the factors activating the migraine. "I want to suggest brief medication trials, for diagnostic purposes."

"No, I don't think so. I don't react well to medications, and besides, I don't like to depend on pills."

I offered further diagnostic studies.

"No, I've had enough testing already."

"How about ten days off work? That might show how much your job contributes to the headaches."

"There's too much going on right now. My next

vacation is six months away."

"A sleep study would be very . . ."

"I sleep fine." rejecting my suggestion in mid-sentence.

I became fascinated. She said "No." to everything. Patients were waiting, but I continued, wracking my brain to see just how many times she could say "No." Finally, "I'm out of ideas. I'm sorry, but I don't think I can help."

She walked out, obviously upset. I knew what she was thinking: "I came all this way, spent all this money, and what did I find? One more doctor who can't fix my headaches."

This story is about a person who tends to say "No." Don't you wonder why a person does this? I think there are some good reasons.

Preference for "No."

Some people like things black or white, yes or no, no shades of gray or in-between. Still others prefer just the no part. You might say it's inborn, one of a person's defining characteristics. Maybe it's part of a strategy, a way to manage life. Whatever it is, if your friends are telling you "Why don't you just say 'Yes.' once in a while?" lookout. You might be one of those "No." kind of people.

About the inborn part: when we say to someone, "You've inherited the completion gene." we're saying that they seem compelled to finish things. A person with this completion trait learns strategies to finish what he or she starts. One way to do that is to take on fewer projects. The more irons you have in the fire, the harder it'll be to finish, and the more frustrated you'll get trying. They've learned to keep it simple; decide what they want to do in life, select just a few things, do them well and "Just say no." to everything else. That way they won't bite off more than they can chew.

In contrast, if you missed out on the completion gene at the moment of conception, you find it hard to finish what you start, but it doesn't matter. In fact you even prefer it that way. If it's not finished, you can still make changes. You like that because it keeps the door open to possibilities.

I'm not sure if the word "no" causes headaches, but I do know that this word can be a baffling reason why they don't get better.

No better

With regard to headaches, the no-trait or personality profile, whatever you want to call it, tends to inhibit or obstruct the discovery of what's causing the headache. Discovery is a process of exploration. How can a person explore; How can we learn anything if we don't try going down a few paths, if we close every door to possibility? "No." stops the search for an answer. Everything about the process of exploring possibilities, including delving into emotions, runs against the grain of a person who does this. More than once I've inquired about stress or emotions, proud of my biopsychosocial approach, only to hear, "I didn't come here for psychotherapy, Dr. Smith!"

Suppose a person's headaches are caused by a lack of restorative sleep and the patient declines a sleep study and a trial of a sleeping pill. Suppose melatonin and herbals have already failed. In a situation like this, there may be no way to prove that sleep is the problem. It's like trying to fix a television set, but you can't use a voltmeter or oscilloscope, and you can't even have the schematic. All I have at my disposal is diagnosis by wit. All I can do is make an educated guess based on experience.

On the other hand, when a person comes with a long list of medications that they've tried and failed, we know quite a bit to begin with. Beyond what the poor response to the medications says, I also know that this is an individual who is willing to try things, who is open to possibility. This person is saying, "Go ahead. Use whatever tools you need to fix me." Then I'm free to pit my experience and my diagnostic skills against the headaches with impunity, that is, without being hampered by "No."

If you're familiar with the Myers-Briggs Type Indicator (MBTI), you will know that I'm speaking of what MBTI calls the Judger or J preference. You might even think less of me for speaking negatively about a person's preference. I know well the merits of the J preference and love them for it. I simply want to point out how the no-word limits possibilities and when it comes to headaches, how it can make them hard to cure. The *"No." in the Air* syndrome is real, and it's a significant cause of headaches that defy a cure; yet I don't see it mentioned in the headache literature. That's why I point it out.

We continue our discussion of saying "No." in Chapter 7 where we see how it allows the patient to stay in control of the visit and, in doing so, stifles the doctor-patient interaction that's essential to finding the underlying cause.

The next story is about a fellow who went to the opposite extreme. He was willing to try anything. Let's see where it got him.

Dopamine Storm

One fellow in particular helped me understand the reason some migraineurs respond to one medication, others to a different medication and why some don't seem to respond at all.

Glass Half-empty: A man in his late 30s came with his father for a one-year history of headaches "day and night." A few times a week they became incapacitating. He went on to say that he had been fighting anxiety, depression and mood swings his entire life. He had trouble sleeping as long as he could remember. His father called him a perfectionist, and on one visit he described himself as a "glass half-empty kind of guy." He was on medications for anxiety and depression; when he tried stopping them, his anxiety and headaches "went through the roof." At times he went into a rage.

Thorough medical and neurological evaluations and a sleep study were unrevealing. By International Headache Society criteria, these might be called chronic daily migraine. I didn't care about the fine points of headache classification. What mattered to me is that he seemed to have some form of migraine driven by strong emotions and lack of sleep, and we needed to understand why that couldn't be fixed.

Medication trials for obsessing and the bipolar/manic trait only made things worse. Anti-epileptic drugs did not help. Inderal in high doses helped a little. The other migraine preventive medications didn't do a thing.

Aside from the longstanding problems, he had been in good health until 10 years earlier when he developed anxiety and depression with OCD tendencies. He came under the care of a psychiatrist at the time, and had been functioning reasonably well on psychoactive medications. A few years before I first saw him, he developed severe mood swings and episodes of rage that became unresponsive to medication, and didn't even respond to a course of ECT (shock therapy).

After nine months, we were getting nowhere. During a particularly scary episode of rage, he went to psych emergency where he signed out against medical advice, as they were about to wheel him off for more ECT. I saw him a few days later and asked myself, "What's staring me in the face here? The biggest things are rage, insomnia and headache."

Then something happened that taught me the meaning of serendipity. A psychiatrist gave me a call about another patient who I had sent to him. "I think she's having a frontal dopamine storm." he said. Frontal dopamine at the D2 receptor creates motivation and get-up-and-go. When frontal dopamine activity is way too high, the get-up-and-go turns into aggression, rage. Suddenly it hit me. "My *Glass Half-empty* fellow . . . that's what's going on with him. He's having a frontal dopamine storm. That's causing his rage."

Rage is an extreme form of the fight-or-flight response. The behavior is largely mediated by adrenaline or, more correctly, epinephrine and norepinephrine. That's why Inderal had some benefit. It blocks the adrenaline effect. Inderal doesn't fix frontal dopamine. Haldol is the drug for that. It turns the volume control down on frontal dopamine. I thought, "If my hypothesis is right, he should respond quite well to Haldol."

A few days later his wife called with a surprising lightness in her voice. "You found it! I've got back the man I married." It was my friend the psychiatrist who found it.

After I hung up, well, the best way to describe how I felt, it felt as if I had just won the lottery. Then I asked myself, "What just happened here?"

> **I had made a discovery. Here was a new way of activating headaches: a frontal dopamine storm stirs up strong emotions; insomnia and the headaches follow.**

I had made a discovery. No, that isn't correct. A psychiatrist and my patient had taught me something. That's a better way to say it.

Haldol isn't a medication for headache; it's an antipsychotic. The fact that a low dose was so dramatically effective proved that excessive frontal dopamine was indeed the activator of his headaches. Not only was it driving his headaches, but also frontal dopamine was behind everything else as well.

Here was a new way of activating headaches: a frontal dopamine storm stirs up strong emotions; insomnia and the headaches follow.

Glass Half-empty was born with strong frontal dopamine chemistry that put him in the middle of a fight-or-flight response much of the time. Who could sleep with those kinds of feelings going on? The strong emotions, lack of sleep, the overpowering adrenaline affect, that's what activated his migraine.

What made this discovery possible? It was just the opposite of saying "No."

What made this discovery possible? It was just the opposite of saying "No."

More about that in Chapter Eight.

————

The stories of serious and baffling headaches leave us with an encouraging thought: When it seems that everything has been done, and there's still no answer, it doesn't mean that we should learn to live with it or be content with treating symptoms. The stories are saying, "Don't close the case. Don't give up. Trust yourself. Find a physician with an open mind, someone who thinks outside the box." The stories urge us to pursue the cause, no matter what, until it's found.

Chapter Six
What I Learned

When a person finally got better, I not only knew the cure. Their story made it clear why the headaches were so incurable in the first place.

It's said that every story has a moral. In each headache success story, there is a lesson about how to do it better, if not a moral. Nevertheless, one case is merely an anecdote that says, "I saw this happen once."

Many cases, however, say something more. Patterns begin to emerge. They may not be proof-positive fact, but at least they say, "Hey. Come over here. Take a look at this."

Let's see what we can learn. What sense can we make of all these stories?

Case after Case

After the *Rice and Water* fellow I set out with the hope of understanding what happens when a person's headaches get better. That's why I chose the success stories. I expected to learn all about the cures for various kinds of headache. I certainly did that.

When a person's headaches showed a dramatic improvement, we had reason to believe that we had found the cure. It's always possible that the headaches would have gotten better on their own as they did in *Sinus Headaches*. Most of the time, though, when the patient got better, it meant that we had found the cure.

When the patient got better, it meant that we had found the cure. Most of the benign headaches proved to be migraine.

Lessons from benign headaches

There were a variety of things my patients did to cure their headaches. Most of the benign headaches proved to be migraine, so treatment largely boiled down to using medications or non-medication approaches to modify the two sets-of-three.

From *Sinus Headaches* we learned that migraine masquerades as many different things: sinus headaches and eyestrain are two of the most common. The story is a warning that diagnosis by assumption is often misdiagnosis. The many different forms of migraine support Edward Liveing's idea that migraine is a family of disorders, a clinical observation that he made in the mid-1800s, which is now confirmed by science.

Migraine masquerades as many different things: sinus headaches and eyestrain are two of the most common.

My own clinical observations carried this a step farther. Although fibromyalgia is not considered a form of migraine, the two are similar in many ways. They both seem to be a state of chronic pain. Although this state of pain may have many causes, lack of restorative sleep appears to be one of the most prominent contributing factors.

The story *Sinus Headaches* is a warning that diagnosis by assumption is often misdiagnosis.

My Story of three years of continual headache led me to believe that mixed-pattern headaches, chronic daily migraine, transformed migraine and tension type headache are, for the most part, just migraine variants in which the neck and scalp muscles are involved. In this theory, muscle pain is one more member of Liveing's family of disorders. Because muscles are involved in this subset of migraine, muscular tension and pain are characteristic features in much the same way that vasospasm is characteristic of basilar artery migraine, another variant.

My Story led me to believe that tension type headache is, for the most part, just a migraine variant in which the neck and scalp muscles are involved.

Real Go-getter, the woman who had basilar artery migraine shows that vasospasm associated with migraine can produce stroke-like symptoms. Vasospasm of this kind accounts for a wide variety of stroke-like neurological symptoms which I called the spectrum of a disorder. When this kind of migrainous vasospasm occurs in the blood vessels of the retina, it produces rapid loss of vision in one eye only. Often called retinal migraine, the vasospasm has even been photographed in a number of cases clearly showing vasospasm in relatively small blood vessels. I went on to assert that any disorder has variants that we can think of as the spectrum of the disorder. Failure to appreciate this idea of spectrum is a significant cause of misdiagnosis. I came to appreciate this notion of spectrum of disease simply by seeing many examples.

Real Go-getter, the woman who had basilar artery migraine, shows that vasospasm associated with migraine can produce stroke-like symptoms.

Failure to appreciate this idea of spectrum is a significant cause of misdiagnosis.

Migraine associated with the manic trait in the case of *Vivacious*, proved to be of utmost importance for several reasons. First, the case illustrated how a medication can be used as a diagnostic molecule to quickly establish the pathogenesis of the headache with a high degree of certainty. In doing so, the case also revealed a subset of migraine, which led to the realization that headache is never the problem. It's only a symptom of an underlying cause. There are many possible underlying causes, that we might think of as subsets of migraine. This one case proved to be of critical importance in much larger ways. We see in Chapter Seven how this case attests to the need for a fundamentally different way of thinking about headache.

The chapter on benign headaches closes with another migraine subset: worry headaches. We see what a complex entity this is, why it's so hard to treat, why diagnostic trials of medication are so important, why non-medication approaches to treatment are crucial to success and why this subset is so common in young people with incurable headache.

Lessons from serious headaches

Those with serious and baffling headaches required a treatment specific to each case.

In the case of *Special Ed* we saw that it is possible to have a headache that looks just like migraine, but in fact it is a headache with migrainous character that is activated by epileptic seizures. I called this *migrainous headache* to make it clear that even though the headache looks exactly like migraine, there's more to it than that. Another way to explain what migrainous means: just because something walks like a duck, quacks like a duck and looks like a duck doesn't always mean that it's a duck. In clinical practice this means that even though a headache meets the migraine definition, it isn't always just a migraine. Clinical definitions have embedded in them a kind of circular reasoning. We start out by saying that some group of symptoms meets the definition of migraine, for example, and since we've defined what we have as migraine, then we don't have to do an evaluation to prove it.

This leads to another flaw in how we think about headache. We often use fancy terms like *primary and secondary headache*, *idiopathic headache* and so forth to hide the fact that we really don't understand what's going on. I suggest using the term *headache of unknown cause*, and just admit our lack of understanding right up front. It's always best to avoid these fancy labels and simply say "I don't understand this." When we do this, we open the door to the search for pathogenesis. This means we have to keep looking until we understand what we're doing.

Swooshing, the case of idiopathic intracranial hypertension,

Vivacious illustrated how a medication can be used as a diagnostic molecule, which led to the realization that headache is never the problem.

Headache in a worrier is a complex entity. It's hard to treat.

Even though a headache looks exactly like migraine, it isn't always just a migraine. Clinical definitions have embedded in them a kind of circular reasoning.

Fancy terms may hide the fact that we really don't understand what's going on. I suggest we simply say "I don't understand this."

shows how easily a serious headache can be missed. In this particular case two emergency department visits concluded "migraine" and dismissed the patient without evaluation. The visits missed the classic red flags of high intracranial pressure and also missed the giveaway to the correct diagnosis: papilledema. To be sure, emergency department physicians must be expected to do an adequate fundus exam on every complaint of headache. It's true as well that emergency departments are not the place to figure out a baffling problem. We need a different setting if we expect to get answers for a diagnostic dilemma.

Swooshing **shows how easily a serious headache can be missed. Red flags point our nose to the answer.**

From *Swooshing* we also saw the importance of recognizing red flags. They point our nose to the answer. Finally, if you're the one with the headache, trust your intuition and find someone who will do a thorough evaluation. Don't go to an emergency department unless it's an emergency.

From *Psychotherapist* we saw how easily herpesvirus infections are overlooked.

From *Psychotherapist*, the woman with facial pain, we saw how easily herpesvirus infections are overlooked. In my experience, they are not only common, they are easily missed, hard to prove, potentially serious and very easily treated. The trick is to make the diagnosis early, so we don't pay the price of continuing pain, what's called postherpetic neuralgia.

It is never good judgement to just pass off an unremitting headache as a psych problem. It needs investigation.

The chapter on serious headaches ended with examples of persistent headaches for which evaluation shows an abnormal finding. We need to understand that sometimes the abnormal finding is indeed the cause of the headache. At other times it is not. As you saw, it can be a real challenge to figure out which is which. It is never good judgement to just pass off an unremitting headache as a psych problem. It needs investigation.

Lessons from baffling headaches

Seven Years of Hell taught me how unaware the general medical community is of migraine variants.

When it came to baffling headaches, *Seven Years of Hell* taught me how unaware the general medical community is of migraine variants, how to confirm the diagnosis and how to treat it. Patient and physician alike may reach a point of desperation with a simple migraine variant that my clinical assistant can diagnose in a few minutes. At a higher level, this case illustrates the importance of being persistent in searching for a diagnosis and how much easier it is to make the diagnosis the next time somebody walks through the door with the problem. With each new cure, I learned something that allowed me to quickly recognize the underlying cause the next time. It also shows how important the correct diagnosis is to the well-being of our patients. The diagnosis and its treatment in this case made it unnecessary to proceed with the cochlear implant she was about to have.

We went on to learn that stubborn headaches can be caused by low oxygen. They're not only common, they are often a mix of chronic lung disease, sleep apnea and carbon monoxide levels from heavy tobacco use, among other things. Once the diagnosis is made, the rest is easy.

A *Preference for "No."* showed how a simple word could account for headaches that no one can fix. Finally we saw in *Dopamine Storm* that the cause of some headaches isn't even in the books. We saw in detail how the cause was discovered. We also saw the incredible cost in time, money and suffering that failure to pursue a diagnosis can have.

> **We went on to learn that stubborn headaches can be caused by low oxygen and how a simple word could account for headaches that no one can fix.**

> **We found that the cause of some headaches isn't even in the books.**

Cure, Cause and Obstacle

Early on, it became obvious that knowing all the cures was not the important thing. That's the easy part. Knowing headache cures is not what we need to know if we are to help a person. We have to understand the *cause* of the headaches. Once we know that, the cure follows right along. It doesn't make sense to treat something when we don't know what we're treating.

As it became apparent that headache is just a symptom of some underlying cause, I realized that treating mere symptoms is a weak form of treatment. It's more effective to address the cause.

> **Knowing all the cures is not what we need to know. We have to understand the *cause* of the headaches. It doesn't make sense to treat something when we don't know what we're treating.**

Headache is never the problem

From the stories of those who succeeded in getting better, it was very clear that we were wasting our time treating the headache. Headache is only a symptom of something deeper, what's known as pathogenesis. The trick was to figure out what that was.

It didn't matter whether it was migraine, a brain tumor, herpesvirus, or a seizure disorder; the headache was never the problem. In every case, there was an underlying cause that had to be found and corrected before the person became well. This principle is just as true for migraine as it is for a brain tumor.

The woman, *Vivacious*, with a bit of the manic trait made it clear how important it is to stay focused on finding the underlying cause and avoid jumping right into treatment. At the end of her last visit with me, her third visit, when her headaches of 20 years

> **Headache is only a symptom of something deeper, what's known as pathogenesis.**

were gone, she made the poignant comment,

> "For the first time in my life, I know what it's like to feel peace inside. If I had this twenty years ago, I never would have been divorced."

Pursuing the underlying cause not only fixed her 20 years of headache, in the snap of the fingers by the way, it also gave her a good night's sleep, a sense of peace she never knew, allowed her to begin the life she wanted, and absolved her of the guilt from what she had done to her marriage under the influence of her birthright: problematic glutamate and GABA receptors. Incidentally, I'll bet it was the vivaciousness that these receptors bestowed that attracted her former husband in the first place. Fixing her headaches did so much more than just fix the headaches.

Cases like this underscore the importance of not treating the headache. It's only a symptom. Staying in diagnostic-mode until we find the underlying cause is what diagnosis really means. It's the best investment if we want to get better.

As I searched through chart after chart, it was no surprise that migraine was the most common kind of headache that I encountered. Half the time the person didn't even realize they were having migraine, usually because they had some migraine variant. They thought migraine was a throbbing, sick headache that makes a person pull the shades and go to bed. They didn't know that their "normal headaches," sinus headaches, eyestrain, "I just feel sick all the time" or some other vague symptom that was hard to get a handle on, was in fact migraine. The first step in getting better was understanding that migraine often masquerades as other things, even puzzling symptoms with no headache at all. When we got to that point, and directed our efforts toward finding the activators, improvement usually followed quickly.

This idea that headache is never the problem has a corollary: diagnosis is everything.

This idea that headache is never the problem has a corollary: diagnosis is everything.

Diagnosis is everything

Knowing all the things that cured headaches didn't seem to help very much. One person with migraine might come back saying, "That doxepin is terrific! My headaches are gone." When I gave doxepin to the next person with migraine, there was no guarantee that it would work.

At one point I stood back from the individual cases to see the big picture. All of a sudden it struck me: "Why, it isn't the treatment that's the problem, it's the diagnosis!" In most cases the person wasn't getting better because there was a flaw in the diagnosis of some kind. An important exception was worry headaches. The problem here *indeed is* the treatment. Even when the diagnosis was spot-on, the treatment was not always highly effective. Worry is simply hard to treat.

Vivacious, is a good example of a diagnostic flaw. She had been on all the migraine medications, and she was still having headaches. When the hypothesis "mild form of mania" came to mind, my next thought was, "If that's the case, Depakote should help." That was easy.

It's possible to have the cure in your hand and not know it. There is a purpose behind every thing I do.

If it's so obvious, then why didn't Depakote help when she tried it years ago? It worked for me. In fact, it was the cure. How is it that in someone else's hands the cure was passed over? This wasn't the first time I'd seen this happen.

It's possible to have the cure in your hand and not know it. I think there's a greater risk of this when a medication trial is done blindly, when there's no hypothesis, no theory of pathogenesis, behind the trial. There is a hypothesis, a purpose, behind every thing I do.

Even before the diagnosis is confirmed, the suspected diagnosis, in a subtle, yet critical way, guides what we do and shapes our interpretation of the patient's response. For example, if the dose is too low or too high, if it's taken at the wrong time of day, an effective medication may have either no benefit or undesirable side effects. The cure might easily be tossed aside!

Obstacles to diagnosis are of critical importance because they force the patient straight into treatment, often treatment of an incorrect diagnosis, that is.

In the light-bulb moment, when the thought "Could this be mania?" popped into my head, I was sure Depakote would work. If it didn't fix the sleep on the first try, I would have varied the dosing until I was certain that it did or did not help. The reasoning behind a medication trial is a critical part of its success.

Assuming you agree that finding the cause of a headache is more important than finding the cure, we must go a step farther.

Defying a Cure - How It Happens

A third theme, the obstacle, is far more important than either cure or cause. Nearly every case sent to me had defied diagnosis. Within each of these stories was another story: the story of how the headaches defied a cure, exactly how it happened.

Obstacles to diagnosis are of critical importance because they force the patient straight into treatment, often treatment of an incorrect diagnosis, that is. If we understand the obstacles to finding the cause in one case, and if we correct them, then we can find the cause more easily in the next case. That translates into fewer people walking around with miserable headaches all the time.

Some cases failed to improve because their evaluation had not been thorough. There were a number of reasons for that. Sometimes it was the patient's fear of testing or fear of doctors. When the patient declines evaluation, we must honor the patient's wishes. It is the patient who has the final say in any evaluation.

> I became fascinated with the many ways these obstacles to diagnosis happened, and even more fascinated by how they were overcome.

I found other forces at work, strong forces, that shaped the extent of evaluation in powerful ways: no way to pay for it, for example. I became fascinated with the many ways these obstacles to diagnosis happened, and even more fascinated by how they were overcome.

Too little time - a matter of resources

Oddly, it seemed that the most common reason some essential finding was overlooked was not because of lack of *diagnostic* testing. The shortcoming is epitomized by a comment made one day by a referring MD, "David I'm sorry for sending these patients, but I just don't have the time to do all the workup they need." I thought, "No need for apology. That's what I do. I figure things out. Referral is a good way for a person to get the evaluation he needs." What he was trying to say is this: When symptoms continue, and we don't know why, the person needs a thorough evaluation. That takes time and effort, often quite a bit more than 15 or 20 minutes.

> When symptoms continue, and we don't know why, the person needs a thorough evaluation. That takes time and effort.

Making a referral to understand a problem you can't diagnose is an efficient use of resources. It's good medical practice in my opinion. It says a lot about the referring physician's quality of care. But what if we do a thorough evaluation and still don't have an answer? Here's how one patient saw it.

> *Back to Square One:* Most of the time a thorough evaluation leads to a definitive diagnosis and the cure; but there are times when we sit there looking at a stack of records, all the labs and scans, and still no answer. All too often at this point, the patient throws his hands up into the air, frustrated, and says something like, "All this work and

still no answer. So, we're back to square one!"

Nothing could be farther from the truth. Another patient in this situation commented, "So, we've learned something!" "Right on!" I thought. Incidentally, he was an MIT-trained electrical engineer.

Even though we have yet to find the answer, we are well beyond square one. Making a diagnosis is like standing at an intersection where one sign points to Boston, another points to Cape Cod and yet another points to Gloucester. When the diagnostic process begins, however, we may see many roads crossing and a dozen signs pointing in different directions. Each negative evaluation narrows the choices back down to a few. We know what the patient does *not* have.

At this point our thinking has moved to a higher plane. If the word I use most is "Why?" then the sentence I use most is "I don't understand this." I lean back in the chair, look at the patient, and that's just what I say.

It's interesting to see what happens next. I sit down with the patient and family, scans in front of us, and together we reconstruct the big picture, an overview or summary. Then we add some details. I might even draw the story out as a timeline. That's when the answers come. It can take an hour or two.

Dr. Joynt's sage advice in *Only 20 Minutes* makes it clear. If we need answers, the history is a goldmine. My friend, the referring physician, was right. It takes interest and often a lot of time to look into things.

Years ago, a wise senior professor and I were discussing how diagnostic errors occur. He said, that "In my experience, errors of omission are more common and more serious than errors of commission." That is, when a patient gets into trouble, more often it's because we did too little. As I write this, I glance at a newsletter from my malpractice insurance carrier. The headline reads, "Case #1: Failure to Diagnose Cauda Equina Syndrome, Case #2: Failure to Refer . . . This is what I mean by errors of omission.

The question should be, "How can we make a thorough workup affordable in time and dollars?"

It takes time and effort to be sure. In cases like this, I don't think the question should be "Do we really need to do all this?" or "How can I get out of doing all this?" I think, there's a better question. "How can we make a thorough workup affordable in time and dollars?"

Diagnosis by assumption

"The doctor pulled a diagnosis out of the air, made a diagnosis by assumption, jumped to conclusions." There are many ways to say it.

There's nothing wrong with making an assumption. I make them all the time. I hypothesize, postulate, theorize and sometimes make a guess. Not only that, I make presumptions, suppositions and I even take things for granted once in a while; but at least I always try to label them as such. I try very hard to never call an assumption a diagnosis. Calling something an assumption means that you're not really sure what it is. It keeps the door open to further investigation and makes one reluctant to treat. "Gee, I don't understand what's going on here. How would I know what to treat you with?"

When we call an assumption a diagnosis, that's how we go wrong, how we wind up treating migraine with an antibiotic and a decongestant.

On the other hand, calling something a diagnosis means that we understand through and through. It stops the investigation and begins the treatment. When we call an assumption a diagnosis, that's how we go wrong. That's how we wind up treating migraine with an antibiotic and a decongestant, and that's why some people never seem to get better.

I find a number of reasons for diagnosis by assumption. Most often it's the wish to practice "cost-effective" medicine or just not enough time or interest to figure things out.

Nonetheless, the approach can be a very effective diagnostic strategy at times. For example, we might say, "This will probably turn out to be migraine activated by your poor sleep. I think I know the cause. Let's treat the cause, and if the headaches go away, we'll have reason to believe that our assumption was correct and we'll have nothing more to evaluate."

There's a subtle problem with this, however: it's another example of circular reasoning. The treatment might cure the symptom, the headache, and leave a potentially serious underlying cause undetected. That might have happened in the case of *Special Ed* if I erroneously thought he was manic and treated him with Depakote. The seizures and headaches would have stopped but I still wouldn't know that he had a seizure disorder behind it all.

Lack of skill

It isn't hard to see that a lack of skill makes error more likely. Two skills are particularly important when it comes to headaches.

Skilled use of novel diagnostic tools: When the scans and bloodwork all come back normal and I'm sitting there looking at the patient only to hear, "So, we're back to square one!" It's tempting to pull a diagnosis out of the air and say, "Well, all the tests are normal, so it's probably your nerves." and send the patient to a psychiatrist. That isn't very satisfying. I feel the same frustration I had that day in the garage, searching for my *Sip of Coffee*.

Instead, as I'm staring at the patient, the first thing I say: "Hmmmm. I still don't understand this. How are we going to figure it out?" Then we talk about diagnostic medication trials, often for just a few days or a week or so. I might suggest using the Wright Brothers' principle or the correlation method to better understand the cause. We talk about it for a while. With the patient's help a good plan usually emerges, but it's a plan to find the diagnosis. It isn't a treatment plan.

> **When we don't have the skill to make the diagnosis, it's tempting to pull a diagnosis out of the air.**

In the case of the *Glass Half-empty* fellow, diagnostic medication trials were of critical importance. My choice of medications was not random or haphazard. With every trial, there was a question that needed an answer. There was a purpose behind everything I did. By the time we did the successful Haldol trial, I was certain that the headaches were not caused by the manic trait, worry, a sleep disorder and half a dozen other things. When all these trials failed, I knew that I was facing something I had never diagnosed before. Without this method of diagnostic medication trials, I would have been just as lost as all the physicians he had seen for years before me. They just sent him to psychiatry where he got ECT. It seemed like no one tried to figure it out.

Psychosocial skills: A second set of skills, psychosocial skills, can make the difference between a good outcome and years of suffering.

Rapid recognition of the worry trait in *Seven Years of Hell* and the manic trait in *Vivacious* allowed me to explore my migraine hypothesis quickly because I knew exactly how these traits activate migraine. Recognizing the worry subset in the first case and the manic subset in the second allowed me to select verapamil as the trial in the first and Depakote in the second. The first medication trial was 100% successful in each case.

> **Psychosocial skills, can make the difference between a good outcome and years of suffering.**

One woman had gone 7 years and the other 20 years with no success. Without a doubt, this tells me that skills in the psychosocial department are lacking in the medical community. If we're wondering why so many people walk around with headaches every day, one answer is staring us in the face right here.

Psychosocial skills help in another critical way. They make it easier to get along with someone, the patient in this case. Let me say it again. A strong mutual trust is essential to solving a problem. Skill in working with different kinds of people is a real asset when we need to build an effective working relationship.

Lack of experience

The greatest shortcoming of learning from experience happens when there isn't enough of it.

MAD Magazine quoted Alfred E. Newman as saying, "The trouble with learning from experience is that you take the test before you get the lesson." There's some truth to that.

When we get a lesson, we acquire knowledge from the experience of others. Learning from experience means that we acquire knowledge from our *own* experience. Some say it's just a matter of preference. There's more to it than that.

The greatest shortcoming of learning from experience happens when there isn't enough of it. A newcomer to a field who has no experience *must* rely on the books and journals and teachers. With time, a person may come to trust his or her own experience more than that of others, especially when he has a lot of it.

In support of the value of experience, it's considered one of the best measures of a training program. The person who has done 10 cataract extractions will probably finish training with less skill than someone who has done 100. As another example, if you've never seen a stenotic basilar artery cause unremitting headaches, you might not recognize the phenomenon when you finish training and go into practice (explanation beyond this text).

You can see that in many cases headaches continued for years because the treating physicians did not recognize the underlying cause or even know how to find it. Here's one way that can happen.

> *Every Excuse in the Book:* When I was in training, one resident seemed to know every excuse for not seeing a patient. If he were called to emergency for a neuro consult he might say, "That's a medical problem. Admit him to medicine, not neurology." . . . "You should be calling psychiatry. Tell them to call neurology if the EEG is abnormal." . . . "Never double-book my clinic patients." (Even though there was a three-month wait to get into the

clinic. Only a few patients ever showed up anyway.)

Those excuses never occurred to me. As far as I was concerned, "Bring 'em on; I'll see anybody, anytime!"

I wound up exhausted with headaches all the time, but I learned a lot. More correctly, my patients taught me a lot. The other fellow, I sometimes wonder how he turned out.

A physician needs more than just experience. He or she needs a *lot* of it. It was experience that taught me how migraine can masquerade as other things and how other things can masquerade as migraine. The idea of masquerade migraine is in the literature, but it wasn't until I saw many cases that I had a feel for the entity. Some of the success stories had defied diagnosis because the doctors before me hadn't seen enough to appreciate the spectrum of the disorder. They had the benefit of the same medical literature that I had. It's just that variations and partial forms of a disorder are much easier to spot when you've seen many of them.

What is it about experience that makes it so valuable? It gives one a *feel* for his area of practice that you can't get any other way. There are three things about this feel that are essential in the practice of medicine: appreciating the spectrum of a disease, having a good feel for liklihoods and recognizing red flags.

> **What makes experience so valuable? It gives one a *feel* for his area of practice that he can't get any other way.**

The spectrum of a disease: It takes experience to appreciate the spectrum of a disease. Remember *Psychotherapist*, the pleasant woman with eye pain for a year due to undiagnosed herpesvirus? A popular and professional website describes the variety of eye problems caused by HSV-1, the cold sore virus, and VZV, the shingles virus. It goes on to say that, except in newborns, neither of these herpesviruses are the HSV-2 herpesvirus that is sexually transmitted and causes genital herpes. Not true. HSV-2 causes eye symptoms that on exam are identical to HSV-1. I've seen it. Experience has taught me to order bloodwork for both HSV-1 and HSV-2 antibodies. If I ordered just HSV-1 antibodies, I would miss every case of HSV-2 eye symptoms that I encounter.

I know this because I have seen many herpesvirus eye cases. If I had only seen one or two cases, or none, I'd be tempted to parrot the website. People might even think that I knew something.

Likelihoods: Experience also creates a good feel for likelihoods. The patient says, "I'm sure it's my allergies." but after

35 years, I know that isn't likely. It sounds more like migraine to me. Another patient is in a panic over the possibility of a brain tumor. I'm thinking, "Very unlikely in this situation."

In the discovery of uncommon and rare causes of headache, experience is essential. For example, temporal arteritis, a vasculitis that's fairly common in those over 60, is easily recognized, diagnosed and treated. Vasculitis in a younger person is uncommon. It takes many forms, and requires experience to recognize and diagnose. I've been in the uncomfortable situation in which someone of less experience calls my evaluation unnecessary or even "inappropriate" only to find Churg-Strauss, a rare form of vasculitis, confirmed by the "inappropriate" evaluation.

In cases like this, it's easy to dismiss something you don't understand as "a psych problem," a conversion disorder or some other emotional problem, until something serious happens. With experience it's possible to see something that's uncommon and immediately know, "This is like no psychiatric problem that I've ever seen." There is something an experienced clinician has that you just can't get from the books and the journals.

Red flags: If a person complains of headache you must get a good look at the optic discs to be sure there's no papilledema, an important sign of high intracranial pressure. There are many, many red flags. Again, it's having the experience of knowing how to use them that counts. It's like learning how to fly. You just can't read the book and expect to take off without crashing.

Every time we solve a problem, we learn something we didn't know before. A problem solved is knowledge gained.

Experience is the best kind of education. Using medications for diagnostic purposes, as disease-defining molecules, and the Wright Brothers principle are things that I learned from experience. Every time we solve a problem, we learn something we didn't know before. A problem solved is knowledge gained. It's a kind of discovery that's not likely to come from a book, and it won't happen at all if you don't persist in your search for the diagnosis.

Unreasonable certainty

In a court of law there's a concept referred to as "reasonable medical certainty." When it's not clear whether a person's loss of vision, for example, was caused by an accident or is part of normal aging, I might be on the witness stand as an attorney asks, "Dr Smith, is it your expert opinion that Mr. So and So's loss of vision was caused by the accident, with reasonable medical certainty?"

In other words, Is it most likely that his loss of vision was indeed caused by the accident?

It isn't hard to see how diagnosis by assumption constitutes what might be called "unreasonable medical certainty." That is, the physician is certain enough to make a diagnosis and treat it, when there is no good basis for such certainty. In the case of *Sinus Headaches*, not only was the diagnosis wrong, it was unreasonably wrong because most of what we call "sinus headache" isn't caused by sinus disease at all. The diagnosis was unreasonably certain, certain beyond what it should have been.

We saw unreasonable certainty play out in the case of *Arachnoid Cyst*. When the epilepsy experts, after five days of EEG monitoring, concluded, "No electrical seizures," I wondered, "Then why does he respond so dramatically to Tegretol?" I sent him to Cleveland where the first thing they did was another EEG, but this time with a sphenoid electrode. In one hour, they confirmed temporal lobe epilepsy.

The experts were "certain" even though their electrode array didn't record from deep structures in the temporal lobes. These deep structures in the mesial temporal lobe, by the way, are the most likely part of the brain to have epileptic seizures, and in this case, the cyst was pressing on that exact part of the brain. I would call the conclusion "No electrical seizures. Here's the name of a pediatric psychiatrist." not just a wrong diagnosis. It was unreasonably wrong because the certainty was unfounded.

I mention this case because I'm sure some would be critical of the way I handled the case of *ventricular asymmetry*. "Why send her out of town and subject her to all that expense and workup when this degree of ventricular asymmetry is common and doesn't cause symptoms? The headaches even had some features of migraine. She certainly proved you wrong when she had her "epiphany"

True. I was aware of psychosocial stressors. In fact, I addressed them on several visits with her husband to no avail. I also knew that headaches that look just like migraine can have a serious underlying cause. At times, her headaches had a sudden onset and offset, the square headache tempo seen in ventricular obstruction. The main reason that I continued the investigation was that I wasn't sure what was going on. Medication trials for worry and emotions had not been effective. I didn't have a diagnosis, so I stayed in diagnostic-mode until I finally did, at least

> Diagnosis by assumption constitutes what might be called "unreasonable medical certainty." The physician is certain enough to make a diagnosis and treat it, when there is no good basis for such certainty. The diagnosis is certain beyond what it should be.

with reasonable certainty.

The problem with unreasonable certainty is that it stops any consideration of other possibilities. "Oh this is such and such. I'm sure. There's no need any more testing." How often I've heard that said in a loud confident voice only to find that that the person didn't have such and such after all.

Unreasonable certainty is a phenomenon for which any physician is at risk, especially physicians in training. With time, I've learned what it means when someone says, "Don't be so sure of yourself." They're talking about unreasonable certainty. Sometimes it's better to just say, "I don't know." and keep searching. A physician I admire said it beautifully: "I enter the room with an open mind." Who knows, you may learn something.

Strongly held beliefs

As members of the human race, we all have strongly held beliefs. They color our perceptions and explain why we do what we do. When it comes to headaches that defy a cure, there's a way they can get us into trouble.

> *Glomming:* A woman with headaches, pain all over, fatigue and the complaint: "I wake up tired," had, so far, failed my efforts to help. One day she returned, elated, with the comment: "I finally found out what's wrong with me! My doctor sent me to a rheumatologist and he said that I have classic fibromyalgia." Then, with a smile, she went on to say, "He told me there's no cure and that I'll just have to learn to live with it."
>
> I sat there, flabbergasted, listening to my patient say how relieved she was, finally, to know what she had. I was witnessing exactly what a person does when he or she doesn't get better. My physician's assistant commented, "She's just glomming on to fibromyalgia. She thinks it's the answer."
>
> She never came back. I guess she took it to heart that she had to learn to live with it.

The rheumatologist gave her a diagnosis that wasn't a diagnosis in the true sense of the word, knowing through and through. I'd call it a pseudo-diagnosis because the understanding was too superficial to help in any real way. What's more, my patient glommed onto the word fibromyalgia and was relieved to have finally found the answer. The belief that she has some untreatable disease with no known cure made her drop the search for the cause.

Today she'd probably be on one of several medications now FDA approved for fibromyalgia. Even with these medications, we don't have what you'd call a high success rate. The FDA website for fibromyalgia *Living with Fibromyalgia* still suggests that we learn to live with it, never stopping to look into why a person is in their state of chronic pain.

In Chapter 3 I mentioned patients who had both fibromyalgia and migraine and how the fibromyalgia improved substantially when we found and treated the underlying cause of the migraine. You've seen many underlying causes of migraine. The most common is lack of restorative sleep, which goes on to create a chronic pain state. This raises the possibility that a lasting, definitive cure for fibromyalgia might be found by using the same approach to finding the underlying cause that I'm suggesting here for migraine.

Glomming onto a diagnosis is similar to pulling a diagnosis out of the air. In each case the search for the correct diagnosis ends.

Glomming onto a diagnosis is similar to pulling a diagnosis out of the air. In each case the search for the correct diagnosis ends. It's just that glomming is based on a strongly held belief, whereas diagnosis by assumption is based on expedience.

Checklist

An important part of taking a history is what's called the review of systems. It's a checklist of trouble signs for each system in the body: heart, lungs, GI tract and so on. I have a similar checklist when a person has headaches. After the patient tells his or her story, I go through the checklist just to be sure I don't miss something.

Here's a simplified version that might help anyone who treats or has headaches. There's no order of priority; they're all important.

Red Flags: There are markers, and there are red flags. Markers are signs or symptoms that help identify the underlying cause. When a marker indicates a potentially serious underlying cause, I call it a red flag. There are many red flags.

Pay attention to anything odd or worrisome about the headaches: a new headache, an increasing pattern or any associated neurological symptom, especially symptoms with a sudden, stroke-like onset. Is there anything unusual: an odd smell that no one else smells (uncinate aura), an audible bruit, cold sores or shingles in the past or a change in behavior?

Migraine Markers: Don't overlook migraine markers. Migraine is a common cause of mysterious symptoms and may occur with no headache at all. The most common migraine markers are a history of headaches of any kind, sensitivity to light, eyestrain, nausea and feeling sick in a vague way that makes it hard to think or do anything.

Sleep: Do you sleep well? If the answer is "Yes," then "Is your sleep restorative? Do you wake up feeling rested or do you want to go back to bed? Do you run tired all day?"

Emotions: Do you feel at peace inside? Are you anxious or angry or sad much of the time? Do you tend to worry about things?

Rebound: Don't overlook alcohol, caffeine and pain killers, or anything that modifies the pleasure-pain system, is habituating, or known to cause rebound headaches. This includes frequent use of marijuana, in my opinion.

Homework: Have you done the necessary soul-searching to be sure that you're not blocking the road to recovery? Ask someone else how you're doing in the anger and no-word departments. Are you open to possibilities? Have you considered the obvious, maybe even what your spouse has been trying to tell you all along?

———

To my surprise, what began as an attempt to find a cure for headaches, wound up as a treatise on the pathogenesis of medical error. If what I found is true, then it's time for a change.

Chapter Seven

The Road Not Taken

What I learned from my patients' stories made it clear that my approach to headache is somehow different. At the core is a different thinking and a different style.

In Chapter One I promised a fresh look at headaches, then asked you to buy into a different approach. Whether you call it a fresh look or a new approach, it adds up to the same thing: taking a different path. In his poem *The Road Not Taken*, Robert Frost describes the process in poetic beauty:

> Two roads diverged in a yellow wood,
> And sorry I could not travel both
> And be one traveler . . .

When it comes to the practice of medicine, choosing a path isn't so simple. Why is one path less trodden? Is it just that we humans are more like sheep than we want to admit. I don't think so. The patients I see are desperate. They're always looking for a new way, something that will help. That goes for the patients and their doctors as well.

If what I've learned about headache from my patients' stories is true, then there's good reason this road is less traveled. The path is no casual stroll. Not everyone seems able to negotiate this one. Some begin, then find they cannot make the journey. They go back and take the easier way.

To walk this road, we need something special. We need two things. One is a style: a particular way that patient and doctor work together. The other is a different way of thinking. Here we begin with the thinking. In Chapter Eight we look at the style.

To walk this road, we need two things. One is a style: a particular way that patient and doctor work together. The other is a different way of thinking.

A Contradiction

Remember the woman named *Vivacious*, who got better when we treated her mild form of the manic trait? A different woman with the same story, returned one day with an intriguing comment: "When I told my PCP how well the Lamictal worked, she just rolled her eyes and said, 'What's Smith doing, treating you with Lamictal? That's not a drug for migraine.'"

Lamictal is not thought to be effective for migraine, but my experience tells me otherwise. Could it be trying to tell us something?

There's a contradiction here. I agree, Lamictal is not considered to be an effective migraine preventative, but my experience tells me otherwise. Is this just some minor inconsistency of no real importance, a fluke? Or could it be trying to tell us something? It's only one case, an anecdote, but let's look into this story carefully and see what we can learn.

The Way It's Done

For migraine, the approach today is straightforward. We listen to the symptoms, do an exam, maybe a scan. If it fits the International Headache Society's (IHS) definition of migraine, we diagnose "migraine" and follow treatment guidelines: First, avoid migraine triggers. If the headaches continue to be frequent and severe enough, we begin one of the preventative medications that have a proven efficacy, in other words, we begin an appropriate medication. That's the way it's done. Most any PCP today would have said the same thing about my choice of Lamictal. It is not an appropriate medication for migraine.

For migraine, the approach today is straightforward. Lamictal is not appropriate.

Knowing what's appropriate: This raises the question: How do we know what's appropriate? A paper given at the American Academy of Neurology (AAN) annual meeting in early 2012 and published in Neurology illustrates the process.

The paper reports a comprehensive review of the headache literature. It was an effort to find the most and least effective medications for the prevention of migraine. The review was done jointly by the AAN and the American Headache Society (AHS) in what is called a meta-analysis, a consensus drawn from many studies. This meta-analysis took into account how well each study was done. The best evidence came from controlled studies that had been done properly and rigorously. So the data was as reliable as one could get. The report concluded that migraine is under-recognized and undertreated and went on to make specific recommendations about preventative medications.

In summary, Topamax and Depakote are two of the most effective migraine preventatives; Inderal is also effective; verapamil has low efficacy and Lamictal is not effective at all. As of April 2012, that's the consensus of the best studies for migraine.

The best evidence from a meta-analysis like this leads to another principle in medicine today: *practice guidelines*. Practice guidelines are recommendations based on a consensus of the experts, the best available evidence. They suggest how to practice in a manner that is considered to be effective and safe. They define what's called the standard of care, in other words, the appropriate thing to do in any particular situation. The American Academy of Neurology has a detailed set of practice guidelines covering the entire field of neurology, including the diagnosis and treatment of headache.

In the practice of medicine today, what "appropriate" means is that we are doing what is generally considered to be the best thing to do. The way we know what's best is to examine well-done studies and use the best evidence to reach a consensus. This leads to practice guidelines which a physician follows with the assurance that he is providing the best care, at least the best care that anyone knows from clinical trials.

This approach is known as evidence-based medicine.

> **What's "appropriate" means that we are doing what is generally considered to be the best thing to do.**

A Different Approach

Evidence-based medicine, as we know it today, did not exist when I began practice in 1977. There were guidelines for good medical care in those days to be sure, but they were informal. Formal or not, there have been guidelines as long as I've been in medicine, and they always have been an important part of what one must learn in becoming a good physician.

As important as guidelines are, they never were enough for me. I needed something more. I never felt comfortable just following what someone else says. It was like following a recipe and not understanding why it was best to do it that particular way. As a medical student and neurology resident, there was always a little voice inside saying, "Is that really true?" In my first year of practice I found that a number of things that I'd been taught were,

> **Guidelines were never enough for me. I never felt comfortable just following what someone else says. I needed something more.**

in fact, not true at all. Things like "If it's pain, it's not MS (multiple sclerosis). Or "If it's a headache every day, it's not migraine." Today we know that these truisms are ridiculously untrue. When we accept as truth everything we're taught, our search for a deeper understanding evaporates into thin air. You can see why an approach like this could never satisfy me. I wanted something more than guidelines. I needed to be allowed to figure things out for myself.

There is good reason for this penchant I have for understanding why.

> **What engineers do is the polar opposite of following. Engineers are compelled to take things apart and understand how they tick.**

What Engineers Do: What engineers do is the polar opposite of following. Engineers are compelled to take things apart and understand how they tick. It's in their genes. When they finally understand how something works, it's clear how to fix whatever's broke about it. Then the engineer is satisfied.

This engineering trait goes right back to my earliest recall. When I was four and five and six, the first thing my father did when he got home from work was to put my toys back together. I didn't play with toys. I took them apart. By the way, if you have a child who does this, you've got a budding engineer on your hands. Understanding how things work is an obsession with the engineering mind. When we don't understand, we feel uneasy. Guess what their favorite question is? "Why." Every other sentence is "Why . . . Why . . . Why . . ." It doesn't matter if you are four or seventy four.

> **The way to make a diagnosis, the way to figure it out when you're dealing with a person is primarily through the story the patient tells.**

At some point in my life, I don't know when, I discovered that there are people in this world who aren't like that. They even like recipes. These individuals are uncomfortable when they don't have rules. They can do something without understanding why; it doesn't seem to bother them. I even wonder if most people in this world are like that.

The answer is in the story: You can understand why I never forgot Dr. Joynt's *Only 20 Minutes* advice. He was telling me right at the beginning of my career that the way to make a diagnosis, the way to figure it out when you're dealing with a person is primarily through the history, the story the patient tells. So that's how, in caring for persons, I've come to take things apart and understand.

What about tools? I used a screwdriver and a pair of pliers as a boy. What would my new set of tools be? As a physician, they became bloodwork, the scans and so on. I even went on to create some new ones: evoked response testing in my early days of practice. Now the tools I find myself using are disease-defining molecules, the Wright Brother's principle and the cross-correlation function. Even with today's high technology, my most important diagnostic tool is still the story the patient tells. As Dr. Joynt said, "The answer is in the history."

In this approach, the evidence comes from talking with individual patients, case studies rather than controlled studies. You might call it narrative-based medicine. For our purposes, I'll call it anecdotal evidence. By this, I mean that how I know what's best to do, comes in large part from talking with the patient. This is the cornerstone of the biopsychosocial approach.

The evidence comes from talking with individual patients, case studies rather than controlled studies. This is the cornerstone of the biopsychosocial approach.

Evidence and Anecdote

Here we see two different approaches to knowing what's best, what's appropriate, as we try to help someone with migraine. One approach has to do what the experts say. The other is to figure out each case as best we can and look for the answers in the pathogenesis. One approach is about following; the other is about understanding. Wouldn't you know, when it came to treating the woman, *Vivacious*, they told me to do opposite things.

How do we explain that? Who's right, evidence-based medicine or anecdote? I'd say that whatever worked was the right thing to do.

Here we see two different approaches to knowing what's best. One approach is about following; the other is about understanding.

Parametric methods: To understand why the conclusions of controlled studies differ from those of the anecdotes, we need to understand the concept of parameters.

To paraphrase the online Wikipedia,[5]

> A parameter is "a limit or boundary." A parametric method of investigation is a study done in a way that limits or restricts what is to be studied and, in turn, limits the results of the study.

For example, when a pharmaceutical company tests a new drug for epilepsy, it may limit the study to individuals 18 to 72. The FDA therefore approves the drug only for individuals 18 to 72.

To understand why the conclusions of controlled studies differ from those of the anecdotes, we need to understand the concept of parameters.

5. Parametric statistics; http://en.wikipedia.org/wiki/Parametric_statistics. Accessed 11/14/2013.

The parameter in this case is an age limit, which means that this study is being done with a parametric method. A non-parametric method would place no limits or restrictions on what is to be studied. The definition goes on.

Most well-known elementary statistical methods are parametric. Generally speaking, parametric methods make more assumptions than non-parametric methods. If those extra assumptions are correct, parametric methods can produce more accurate and precise estimates. They are said to have more statistical power. However, if those assumptions are incorrect, parametric methods can be very misleading. For that reason they are often not considered robust. On the other hand, parametric formulae are often simpler to write down and faster to compute. In some, but definitely not all cases, their simplicity makes up for their non-robustness, especially if we take care to examine the method carefully for underlying assumptions.

The evidence of evidence-based medicine mostly comes from parametric studies. This means that assumptions built into these methods could give rise to misleading conclusions.

The evidence that forms the foundation for evidence-based medicine mostly comes from parametric studies. This means that assumptions built into these methods could give rise to misleading conclusions.

Non-parametric methods: The most non-parametric method that I know is the history of the patient's illness. A good history makes no assumptions. That isn't perfectly true. The story is colored by the perceptual distortions of the patient, and those of the doctor for that matter. I think you understand what I'm trying to say. A good history is much less restrictive and is open to more possibilities than a controlled study could ever be. It simply listens to what the patient is trying to say and listens with an open mind. Besides, taking a history is cheap and quick, 20 minutes instead of the years it might take to complete a study.

A parametric method is like an interrogation. A non-parametric method is like an open-ended interview. Both are narrative methods, but the stories they tell can be quite different.

There's a simple way to think of the difference between parametric and non-parametric methods. A parametric method is like an interrogation. It asks a question and gets an answer. A non-parametric method is like an open-ended or non-directive interview. It begins with something like, "So tell me all about . . . " Then the interviewer just listens without one more word. He asks questions, the parametric part, but only at the end, after the patient has told the story without any limit put on what he has to say. A parametric study is an interrogation; a non-parametric study is an open-ended interview. Both are narrative methods, but the stories they tell can be quite different.

I think you can see where this is going. I'm wondering, "Does evidence-based medicine draw a different conclusion because the evidence, upon which it is based, comes from parametric studies which make assumptions that are not made when we take the patient's history? Is that why the studies say that Lamictal doesn't help migraine while the anecdotes say the polar opposite?"

Even though the notion of parameters explains why the two approaches come up with different conclusions, we still don't know which one is right. When the next person comes in with migraine, do I consider Lamictal or don't I?

The assumption: The studies that found Lamictal is ineffective as a migraine preventative assumed that migraine is one thing: migraine. They measured the efficacy of various preventatives for migraine-as-a-whole without regard for subsets.

What I call the anecdotal approach found that it doesn't make sense to treat the migraine because it's only a symptom of an underlying cause. There are many underlying causes. I know this because that's what the patients' stories tell me. In the case of *Vivacious*, not only did the history reveal the presence of an underlying cause, it told me exactly what the cause was.

The history defines the pathogenesis of the migraine in most cases. If a patient's headaches go away when I treat the underlying cause, I have good reason to believe that what I presumed to be the pathogenesis is, in fact, correct. It's no surprise that my treatment was different and used medications not even considered useful for migraine. That's because I wasn't treating migraine. I was treating manic illness, worry, a frontal "dopamine storm," anything but migraine.

True, if you treat migraine as a whole without regard for underlying cause, Topamax helps the most and Lamictal not much at all. It is also true that if you find and treat the underlying cause, you will find a number of effective medications not on the list of migraine preventatives. I maintain that they will be highly effective because they are directed to the pathogenesis, not the symptom.

Let me say this again in different words. If you do studies to measure how effective various medications are in preventing migraine and if you do these studies without taking into account

> **Even though the notion of parameters explains why the two approaches come up with different conclusions, we still don't know which one is right.**

what is causing the migraine, they will show what the AAN/ASH meta-analysis found: Topamax is effective and Lamictal is not. However, if you first talk to the patient, find the cause of the migraine and treat that, you find what I am saying here: The treatment is more effective when it's done this way and even includes medications not considered helpful by the first approach. To say it simply, if you treat without regard for the underlying cause, you will get the meta-analysis result. If you treat the underlying cause, not the migraine, I maintain that you will have a better result. Failure to treat the underlying cause also explains why the efficacy of the meta-analysis approach is not very high.

Both conclusions are true. It's just that the conclusion from the controlled studies is irrelevant.

So both conclusions are true. It's just that the conclusion from the controlled studies is irrelevant because anecdote shows that all migraine is not the same. Experience has taught me that it's best to match the treatment to the *cause* of the migraine.

Stand back for a minute and take a look at the big picture here. Taking a history, a non-parametric method that makes no assumptions, allowed me to realize that I was asking the wrong question: "What's the cure?" Not only that, it pointed my nose to what the important question really was: "What's the cause?"

Controlled studies, parametric methods, ask a question and stick to it. They have no way to tell if it's a relevant question or not. That's how a study can be misleading. It's possible for a controlled study to get evidence that's true, but irrelevant.

Evidence from controlled studies can be thought of as a consensus of the experts.

Evidence from controlled studies, as I said, can be thought of as a consensus of the experts. Here's something else to consider:

A lesson from relativity: In the practice of medicine today consensus is the gold standard, even to the point of penalizing someone who thinks differently. However, there are ways to understand this amazing world we live in, other than by consensus. As I reflect on all this, I'm reminded of an important event in the history of our species.

However, there are ways to understand this amazing world we live in, other than by consensus.

Einstein: Imagine you're a physicist in the early 1900s, and you are trying to understand how things like the speed of light and energy and matter all fit together. So you call together the best physicists of your time: Max Planck, Niels Bohr, Ernest Rutherford, Werner Heisenberg, Erwin Schrödinger, Wolfgang Pauli and Paul Dirac, all brilliant physicists, no question about that, all Nobel Laureates - the cream of the crop. You get them talking and summarize what they say with a consensus statement. Would that give you the best insight into the question at hand?

Absolutely not. It took an Albert Einstein to put it all together; but even he freely admitted that e = mc² and all that goes along with it was only a theory. Einstein himself made the comment, "Proving it is up to someone else."

Evidence-based medicine and my anecdotes appear to lead in different directions Could we combine the two in some way to achieve the best of both possible worlds?

Thinking like an engineer, I found a problem with "the way it's done" today. Evidence-based medicine and my anecdotes appear to lead in different directions when it comes to patient care. An interesting question follows: Could we combine the two in some way to achieve the best of both possible worlds?

The Best of Both Worlds

In the future, I'm sure we will have a way to erase a person's susceptibility to migraine. Like my father who never had one, it will be as if we were born without migraine genes. Then we can worry as much as we want, sleep as little as we want and drink all we want, and never get a headache. Maybe we're better off with our migraine. At least it keeps us on the straight and narrow.

For now though, it looks like we're stuck trying to find better ways to understand headaches and get rid of them. I propose an approach for your consideration, a way that combines the best of controlled studies with the best of anecdote.

The best part of controlled studies is that they allow us to say, "I know this." or "I know that." They allow us to know something with reasonable certainty, provided we ask the right questions. If we ask the wrong questions or do the study improperly, we may know something with a high degree of certainty, but wind up with a strong directive to "Do it this way." which might not be the best way. Following an ill-conceived study with erroneous conclusions, we become the blind leading the blind. Who knows where that will take us? Ultimately it's the patient who pays the price.

The best part of anecdote is that it encourages us to take something apart and figure out how it works without making assumptions that put limits on what we might discover. Anecdote encourages us to search for underlying cause. Once we discover an effect, anecdote doesn't tell us how significant it is or even if we've interpreted our findings correctly. We need studies to do that.

Anecdote has the power of generating innovative theories about how things work. Controlled studies can prove or disprove the theories to some degree. The anecdotes help generate the relevant questions and the studies give the answers with a degree of certainty.

A Proposal: My proposal is this: Use anecdote to generate new theories of how things work and to raise questions that have relevance. Then use studies to prove or disprove these theories and questions.

> Anecdote has the power of generating innovative theories about how things work. Controlled studies can prove or disprove the theories to some degree.

Like taking a patient's history, the order is important. The open-ended, non-directive (nonparametric) part goes first, the interrogation (parametric part) is second. We have to find the important questions before we try to prove them.

In concept it's a simple approach, but it's necessary. Without a marriage of study and anecdote, I'm afraid we will be treating our patients without an understanding of what we are treating for a long time to come.

Here's an illustration of how this marriage might work. I have found subsets of migraine that are activated by specific underlying causes. They are, for the most part, easily treated. Mania-activated migraine is the subset into which the vivacious woman falls.

I have also found that when we finally identify and treat these underlying causes, headaches that have been refractory to treatment finally resolve. Clinical experience is the basis for these findings, so my evidence is anecdotal. Some of the causes may be unusual, but others occur often enough to form patterns that are easily recognized. Nevertheless, the notion of subsets is a hypothesis, a theory that needs proof.

> Without a marriage of study and anecdote, I'm afraid we will be treating our patients without an understanding of what we are treating for a long time to come.

Therefore, I propose that controlled studies be done to prove the following: when a group of migraineurs is divided into subsets according to the underlying cause, and when this underlying cause is treated, the efficacy of treatment is significantly better than when we treat the group as a whole without regard to underlying cause as it's done today.

Studies of this kind, if done properly, would add credibility to the importance of identifying migraine subsets.

. . . and a caution: If there is to be a marriage of study and anecdote, it must be a marriage in spirit, not just a formal agreement between two parties who have little regard for one another. Otherwise, I fear that we'll be generating more misleading studies. Let me show how this might happen.

Imagine someone says, "Okay, Smith, I'll put your theory to the test." They design a rigorous study to prove or disprove whether or not there is a subset of migraineurs with a subtle form of the manic trait who don't sleep and therefore get headaches. So they select a few anecdotists and a psychiatrist or two to oversee the study. Chances are, even if the anecdotists believe in the importance of a good history, if they don't have the skill to recognize a subtle form mania, the study probably will end with an erroneous conclusion.

It's likely to conclude that not only is the Lamictal response much less than Smith believes; it's hard to even find the kind of cases that he's describing. The conclusion would be erroneous because the recognition of subtle forms of mania is a skill unto itself. So the study might erroneously label individuals who don't have the brain chemistry of mania as "manic." A person who doesn't have the glutamate/GABA abnormality won't respond to Lamictal. Others who have the manic trait may be overlooked because it was too subtle to be recognized. So there I am continuing to treat people successfully with Lamictal while evidence-based medicine says that I'm wrong.

I'm not saying that this kind of error might occur. I'm certain that it will occur unless the study is specifically designed to prevent recognition errors of this kind. Why am I so sure? Because I have seen many of these cases, individuals who have gone years with insomnia and headaches before someone finally recognizes and treats the manic trait. I'd even say that failure to recognize the trait is more common than not. It's the reason so many don't get better.

Again, I'm using anecdote, in this case, to make the assertion that the manic trait is under-recognized. Again, I haven't proven a thing. Nonetheless, it's an observation, an important observation that might dramatically alter the design of the study and the correctness of its conclusions.

No Fluke

Some things we will never know by doing studies and taking a consensus.

Petri Dish: In 1928 when Alexander Fleming, by chance, looked into a discarded Petri dish and saw a ring of no bacterial growth where a fungus had contaminated the culture, he didn't toss the culture and say, "Just a fluke." Curious, he looked into it and discovered penicillin. That trivial observation ushered in a whole new age of medicine. Now a person seldom dies of infection that had taken the lives of countless men, women and children in the time before antibiotics.

While the case of *Vivacious* may not have the profound significance of the discovery of penicillin, it was certainly not a fluke. Her story is a highly significant piece of evidence. A mere anecdote has detected a flaw in the foundation of evidence-based medicine: It makes too many assumptions.

Specifically, this case and many like it suggest that, with regard to migraine, the headache is not the problem and that it doesn't make sense to treat the headache with preventatives. It also explains why: because there is an underlying cause that begs to be treated. In this sense, treating migraine is no different from treating the headache caused by a brain tumor. You don't treat the symptom. You treat the cause of the headache and the symptom goes away.

A mere story has shown a contradiction between evidence and anecdote. It's calling for a change in our thinking.

I began this chapter saying, "It's only one case, an anecdote, but let's see what we can learn." To say it differently: "Yes, *Vivacious* is just a case, but she is also part of a pattern that I've see in others." Identifying the subsets of migraine will be our first step in redirecting our attention from treating a symptom to searching for the underlying cause. Beyond migraine, I believe this approach will be a major contribution to the understanding and treatment of headaches of all kinds.

Like Fleming's Petri dish, the story of *Vivacious* has shown a contradiction between evidence and anecdote. It's no fluke. The story is saying that we must find and treat the underlying cause. It's calling for a change in our thinking.

———

Here we have a different approach, a road less traveled, a prime example of Apple Computer's slogan "Think Different." Have you ever wondered how medical care might look today if Steve Jobs had applied his "think different" philosophy to medicine instead of computers?

Chapter Eight

A Matter of Style

The second part of this different approach is a different style in the way that patient and doctor work together.

In this chapter, we consider the style in which patient and doctor work together. What do our stories say about a relationship between patient and doctor that promotes discovery. I want to say something to the patient and something to the doctor.

To the Patient

It's surprising how well most visits go and how much progress we make in situations that are very difficult for a person who's under the weather with headaches. It's remarkable to see how positive most people are when I'm trying to help. It's a credit to the patient.

However, there are always visits that don't go well. From those unsettling visits, I've found three things that, as the patient, you must keep in the front of your mind: gratitude, insight and saying "Yes." They shape the process of discovery and healing profoundly. I want to explore just what it is that goes on in a person's head when the discovery process isn't working and how it's different when we find success.

Drawing from the writing of Henri Nouwen,[6] I think of them as *movements* that a person makes in life.

The movement from anger to gratitude

Returning to **Glass Half-empty**, he was in agony with what seemed to be an impossible problem. He was in pain, his emotions were in turmoil beyond comprehension and his family was at wit's end; yet he got better. How did that happen?

I want to explore just what it is that goes on in a person's head when the discovery process isn't working and how it's different when we find success.

6. Nouwen H. *Reaching Out. 1975 Doubleday, Garden City.*

In retrospect, I didn't even have his cure in my bag of tricks when he first walked in the door. We had to discover something new. What was it that allowed all this to happen? What was the magic? The way that emotions played out during his visits was particularly instructive.

Anger: He came for help with his headaches, but his visits were all about anger. Do you ever wonder why we have emotions? I believe we have emotions to make things happen. They accelerate and intensify how we respond to what's going on about us.

For example, the emotion we call joy rewards us so that we try to make whatever just happened, happen more. Joy says, "I want more of that!" Joy conditions us to do whatever it takes to get more of what we want.

Grieving, on the other hand, does just the opposite. It makes us do certain things and not do other things that make whatever we don't want to happen, happen less. Joy is the emotion that motivates one of the most important dimensions of life: attachment. Grieving is our response to losing that attachment. It's most intense when we lose a loved one.

Two other emotions, fear and anger, intensify our response to a threat. They are the emotions of the fight or flight response, which is mediated in large part by adrenaline. If a saber-tooth tiger is about to attack, fear would make a primitive man run much faster than he would without the emotion. Fear, which also takes the form of anxiety or terror, has survival value.

On the other hand if the tiger is about to attack his mate or child, he feels a different emotion, rage. It's milder form is anger. It's a natural response to feeling victimized; it intensifies our wish to do harm in return. That's why it's so scary when someone directs their anger toward us. That's why it hurts so much when we're on the receiving end. We feel that they want to harm us.

Most anger that we as humans experience proves to be a disaster. There's headache, and there's headache in an angry person. From the point of view of someone who's trying to help, they are two very different things. A person may come for one problem, headache, but then we have two problems, the one he came with and the anger. What's more, the anger makes it hard to figure out the first problem because it's in control of the situation. When that happens, the chance of a good outcome plummets. Sometimes I just have to say, "Let's push the emotions aside and focus on the

> **Anger is a natural response to feeling victimized; it intensifies our wish to do harm in return. That's why it's so scary when someone directs their anger toward us. We feel that they want to harm us.**

headache for now."

> *I Didn't Like You:* One day when a patient returned for a follow-up visit, the first things she said was, "I didn't like you on the last visit, Dr. Smith."
>
> I understood. She had been abused as a child. As often happens when someone is abused during the formative years, the child learns to control his or her world by becoming ill, especially ill with pain. As a patient, she pressured me for narcotics. She was whining and dependent and not getting better. The behavior pushed one of my buttons.
>
> I didn't raise my voice or do anything overtly angry at the time, but my tone of voice did change and she picked up on it immediately.
>
> She was right. I was angry. So I gave her a sincere apology. "I'm very sorry for that and I apologize."
>
> There was an immediate sense of relief in the air, and we were able to re-establish a good working relationship. The last thing that she did on leaving that day was to give me a big hug.

The Grimm's fairytale, *The King of the Golden Mountain*, shows how damaging anger can be in a relationship.[7] The story begins with a wealthy man who has lost his fortune. All that's left is a field where he meets an evil dwarf. The dwarf tricks the man into giving up his son in exchange for a fortune greater than the one he lost. Trying to comfort his father the boy says, "Don't worry Father, the dwarf has no power over me." His son is sent away. On his journey he comes across a snake.

> "The snake, however, was an enchanted maiden, who rejoiced when she saw him and said, 'Are you coming, my redeemer? I've been waiting for you the twelve years . . .'"

He breaks the spell, they marry and live happily together as the King and Queen of the Golden Mountain. She bears a "fair boy." Eight years later, in a fit of anger, he lops off the heads of everyone he holds dear. As the story ends, there he is, the King of the Golden Mountain, alone.

The evil dwarf represents anger. When the boy said to his father, "Don't worry Father, the dwarf has no power over me." he could not have been more wrong. Anger has an incredible power

7. Translation by Magoun FP, Krappe AH *The Grimms' German Folk Tales*. Southern Illinois University Press, 1960, Carbondale and Edwardsville.

over us. It takes us down a path to a place we don't want to be.[8]

If I had said to my patient, "Me? I wasn't angry. You must be mistaken." then I don't think our relationship would have recovered. Just saying that anger doesn't exist doesn't make anger, and the power it has over us, go away.

Here's the important thing: Anger loses its power over us when we lay the excuses aside, admit that we are angry and simply offer our sincere apology. Fortunately, I could recognize my anger and say, "I'm sorry." That put the evil dwarf right out there in front of us, so we both could look him square in the eye. That's what redeemed our relationship.

> **Anger loses its power over us when we lay the excuses aside, admit that we are angry and simply offer our sincere apology.**

Why is anger so harmful when it finds its way into a relationship? It seems to make intimacy impossible. When there's a good feeling going on, I can greet a person I've never seen before, and five minutes later we're talking about things that are very personal. "Gee, I've never even told my husband that!" We may need to get to that level if the visit is to be worthwhile, if it's to be of any help.

When anger is in the air, no matter what the reason, we can't get close, let alone solve a problem together. One thing is sure: It's hard to trust someone who's angry with me because anger is the emotion that says, "I want to harm you." We don't feel safe.

In personal relationships anger does something much more insidious but equally damaging. It has to do with recognition. When we recognize someone who's part of our life, the process in our brain goes something like this: "Oh, I know that person. I know that face. I know that voice." But there's one more thing that happens. The important part of recognition is this: That physique, that face, that voice is connected with a feeling. Your brain says, "That physique, that face, that voice, *that feeling I have* . . . Oh. That's my wife!"

> **When anger is in the air, we can't get close, let alone solve a problem together.**

If head injury or stroke disconnect the recognition from the feeling, the person will say, "She looks and talks just like my wife, but that isn't my wife. She's an imposter." He says that because he doesn't have the feeling inside that he usually gets from his wife.[9]

Now, imagine what anger does in a relationship when there's no head injury or stroke. Every angry encounter creates an increasingly strong, painful association with the person. You can take it from there.

8. My interpretation.

9. Known as the Capgras phenomenon.

Gratitude: So what was different about *Glass Half-empty*?

What was going on in his head that allowed us finally to find the answer to his peculiar problem?

He was born angry, very angry. That's how his frontal dopamine circuits were wired. We had many visits, many unsuccessful visits. That would have made just about anybody angry. How could this man *not* have directed his frustration and anger toward me?

I know the answer to that question because I felt it, clearly. At the end of every visit he looked me in the eye and, in the most genuine way possible, said how much he appreciated my efforts. Can I tell you how good that felt? Appreciation was the magic that made everything turn out well. Gratitude is an antidote for anger. It brings two people together, allowing them to form a bond. We became close during those visits. More than once he said how much he trusted me. How could we trust someone if we're angry with them? Our anger shows that we feel victimized, just the opposite of what this fellow was feeling.

What was different about *Glass Half-empty*? What was going on in his head that allowed us finally to find the answer?

In Italy, when someone does something nice for you, a person expresses gratitude by saying "Grazie." I means "Thank you." Grazie comes from the Latin root gratia, which means gratitude. There's another word derived from the same Latin root. It's the word grace. What this says to me is that a very long time ago someone realized that gratitude is the essence of grace. That's what the *Glass Half-empty* fellow had. His magic was grace. I'm left with a great deal of admiration for that man. His gratitude allowed him to hold onto his sanity, even when the chemistry in his brain was trying to make him do just the opposite.

At the end of every visit he looked me in the eye and, in the most genuine way possible, said how much he appreciated my efforts.

Isn't that amazing? Here we see how a matter of the spirit, gratitude, prevented anger from taking control and overcame the effects of a chemical disorder of the brain.

If it sounds to you like I'm anger-bashing, I apologize for that too. I realize that anger has a useful function. After all, that's why we have the emotion. It's there for a reason. It's there to intensify our response to a threat and things worse than just a threat, things like the moral outrage of World War II. So anger, like worry, has survival value. It's not meant to be used against loved ones, especially your spouse and your children. If you can keep it out of your relationship with your doctor as well, you'll have a much better chance for a happy ending. This one change can make the difference between success, or not.

Gratitude is an antidote for anger.

If anger is the emotion we use best, we might learn something from my friend *Glass Half-empty*. If you want to get better, first, you'll need to learn something about gratitude.

The movement from denial to insight

A spouse may sometimes shed light on a puzzling headache.

Problem at Home: Years ago I saw a pleasant young woman who had a migraine headache every day. She was a secretary in a stressful, fast-paced office and required Imitrex every day just to get by. I tried many things over a few months, including Imitrex withdrawal to see if she had a form of analgesic rebound. I got nowhere.

As she was leaving one day, I said, "You know I've never met your husband. How about coming back with him next time?"

A worried look came to her face. "You want to see me with my husband? Why do you want to see my husband?"

"Well, you know, it gives me a different perspective on things. Maybe we'll learn something. We haven't made any progress in almost three months now. You still get a headache every day and you're using way too much Imitrex."

Indeed she returned with her husband. They sat to my left side. I was behind my desk. About five minutes into the visit, I was calibrating with her husband with small-talk, when I noticed a tear running down her cheek. I turned to her and said, "Whoa, what's that about?" Her husband looked at her, saw the tear, turned his back, crossed his arms and said, "Look Doc. I tell her 'You want a divorce? Get one!'"

There was a long silence. I didn't know what to say. I don't remember what happened after that, only that it was a short visit.

> **It isn't enough just to stop denying what's obvious. We have to go to the opposite extreme. Stand back, and keep asking "What's really going on here?"**
>
> **Taking an honest look at ourselves goes a long way toward finding the cure.**

After they left, I just stood there dumbfounded, asking myself, "On the first visit, why didn't she just say, 'Look, I work hard all day at a stressful job, and when I go home, it isn't a happy home. It's even more stressful there.'"

I don't know who was right and who was wrong. Maybe nobody was wrong. I'm simply trying to tell a story that taught me a lesson: Don't ignore the obvious. Because of this principle, the best visits are usually the visits with family.

It's so hard to see ourselves through the eyes of others because everything we do seems so right and normal. You can see this at work in the stories of *Connoisseur*, *No Reason Why*, *Asymmetric Ventricles* and *Closing Doors*.

If you want my advice, it isn't enough just to stop denying what's obvious. We have to put our intuition to work and go to the opposite extreme. Stand back, open your eyes and keep asking yourself "What's really going on here? What's really going on?" You might even try asking your spouse.

Taking an honest look at ourselves goes a long way toward finding the cure.

The movement from "No" to "Yes."

In Chapter 5, *"No." in the Air* made it clear how closing doors by saying "No" hampers the search for the cause, intimidates the physician, stops the back and forth conversation and takes away one of the most powerful diagnostic tools, medication trials. Saying "No." to things limits a person's life. That's one thing you don't want if you're going to find the underlying cause of a problem. How is it different when a person succeeds in becoming well?

> **Saying "No." to things is one thing you don't want if you're going to find the underlying cause of a problem. Here the control stays with the patient.**

The most striking difference is that patient and doctor are tossing around one idea after another. They are considering many different possible causes and how to confirm or exclude each one. Patient and doctor are passing *control* back and forth. Anything is up for consideration. No limits. Nothing is sacred or untouchable.

This interaction has a very different feeling from the conversation with a no-kind-of-person. Here, the control stays with the patient. The best way to illustrate this kind of successful problem-solving is with a comment made by a relative of mine.

> *All of Us:* Craig, my brother-in-law works for a pharmaceutical company. He manages the drug reps who call on physicians. I was at a fundraiser for multiple sclerosis some years ago when I struck up a conversation with a drug rep. Without knowing that he was my brother-in-law, she began to talk about Craig. "I used to work for him. He's the best boss I've ever had, by far!"
>
> When I asked what made him such a good boss, she said something like, "He listens." I still didn't understand what it was that was so different about Craig, but I did know that I wanted some of whatever he's got.
>
> A few weeks later when the family got together for

> **There's an old saying: "None of us is as smart as all of us."**

the holidays, I mentioned what the rep had said. "What's your secret, Craig?"

"Oh it's simple. There's an old saying: 'None of us is as smart as all of us.'"

Craig's approach is much different from what you might call control-management, in which the boss makes the decisions and hands them down. That keeps the boss in control, but it isn't the best way to solve a tough problem.

I've taken Craig's advice to heart. He's right. When we put our heads together, none of us has a good solution at the start. Then the ideas start to bounce back and forth from person to person. It's amazing how quickly a good plan just seems to appear, something none of us would ever have imagined. An approach like this honors what each one of us is trying to say.

"Learning to speak the language of possibility." It means giving up some control and trying some new things.

If you have headaches and can't seem to find the answers you need, then take a day and count how many times you say, "No." or what amounts to "No." Perhaps the no-word is in control. You may just need some new words in your vocabulary, some yes-words. One of my mentors calls it "learning to speak the language of possibility." It means giving up some control and trying some new things.

Sometimes a door gets stuck. It may be hard to open, but how can we get anywhere in our search for some answers, if we don't open some doors and look behind them?

To the Doctor

"OK." you say, "That's what I have to do. But how do I find the other part, the right doctor?" Before a patient tells me what he thinks a doctor should do, I sometimes hear about what the last doctor didn't do. Although it's said in many ways, most of the complaints fall into three areas: 1) "He didn't listen, had his mind made up, was dismissive." 2) "He didn't look into things, he just pulled a diagnosis out of thin air." and 3) "He wasn't very friendly."

Maybe if we look at the opposites of these, we could gain some insight into how the doctor's part could be better.

Although I'm speaking to the doctor now, the next three items should help the patient size up the doctor side of the equation. In other words, is this a person who's likely to help?

The movement from speaking to listening

When someone listens to me, I sense that the person values what I have to say. It's a bonding experience. Duffy is a good listener.

> *Duffy:* If I had to say one thing about my dog Duffy and me, it's that we have bonded. I know this because, on my end, I like to be with him. Every time I look at him, I say to myself "You are beautiful." He's a golden retriever, so it isn't hard to feel that way.
>
> I know we're bonded on his end because he waits for me at the door. And the first thing he does when I come home from work is stand up and put his arms (front legs) around me. Then he looks me straight in the eye with that beautiful dog face of his and licks my face a few times.
>
> We're bonded all right. There's no question about that. My wife Mary just looks on and shakes her head.

Duffy's vocabulary isn't more than a handful of words, so much of what I say, he just doesn't get. The brain that he was born with didn't come with the ability to decode English. I know he listens because when I talk to him, he just sits there perfectly still, looking me straight in the eye. You're probably thinking, "Whoa, this guy's off his rocker. I better close this book right now and give it to Goodwill." Listen on.

The point I want to make is that even without understanding the words, Duffy truly listens. There's no question about that. I feel it; just by the way he sits there without interrupting as he looks straight at me. Maybe he doesn't get the part where I tell him how to be a transcendent canine, but he does understand the important part by how I talk to him. My tone of voice is saying, "You know old fellow, I really love you." That's what he likes to hear because that's what's important to him. Isn't that what's important to every one of us?

After writing these few paragraphs, I said to Duffy, "You're in my book, you know." He doesn't even know what a book is, other than something to chew on. What's it matter anyway? What matters is "Do you love me?" He's just a dog, but he knows what's important.

Whether I'm talking to a patient or Duffy, it's the same. Feelings transpersonalize, and they do so in a powerful way. Agree

> **When someone listens, I sense that the person values what I have to say. It's a bonding experience.**

> **My tone of voice is saying, "You know old fellow, I really love you." That's what he likes to hear because that's what's important to him. Isn't that what's important to every one of us?**

or not, how well I listen to a person is the first step in forming a bond. It says "I want to hear about your world." If we listen in the right way, it says, "I care about you." in one of the most genuine ways possible. The feelings that patient and doctor have as they talk back and forth are a confirmation check on whether they are together or not.

I could go on and discuss how non-directive history-taking is better than interrogation and how the response to what a person says needs to be congruent, but they aren't the important things about listening. The important thing is this. Listening to a person says "I care about you." in one of the most genuine ways possible.

Duffy understands this. I wish more humans did.

The movement from assuming to understanding

In the office with a patient sitting in front of me, I'm quite aware that I am serving the interests of two parties. One is whoever pays for the evaluation. The other is the patient who receives its benefit. Every physician weighs this cost and benefit when deciding to recommend a test or not.

The case of *Sinus Headaches* shows how costly diagnosis by assumption can be in the long run. In my opinion, the first physician who sees a person for sinus headaches must do an eye exam to be sure there's no papilledema and order an MRI scan of the head. This is the starting point for any kind of headache. No papilledema means that the intracranial pressure is most likely normal. Usually the scan is normal as well. At the outset, we know there's no sinus disease and no brain tumor. We've ruled out most of the other serious causes of headache. Bloodwork rules out most underlying medical problems that cause headache.

If the doctor begins with an evaluation rather than a prescription, he knows many things for which he doesn't have to write a prescription.

Many doctors don't do this. It's considered "too much testing." Most of the time when a person first presents with sinus headache, the doctor just prescribes an antibiotic, when most of the time sinus disease is not the cause. This is my experience. If what I say is true, wouldn't it make more sense to order the tests on the first visit? The MRI doesn't have to be expensive. A brief protocol is quite adequate in this situation.

If the doctor begins with an evaluation rather than a prescription, he knows many things for which he doesn't have to write a prescription. You, the patient, don't have to waste time and money on antibiotics, unhelpful follow-up visits, an ENT consult and possibly an emergency department visit in the middle of the night. With possibilities narrowed down considerably, doctor and patient can focus on what's left. The patient is thinking, or even says out loud, "Here's a doctor who's really doing something." They appreciate the good care, and everybody's better off in the long run.

The cost of misdiagnosis can be unbelievably high and often extends over years, as you've seen with some of the cases here, not to mention the cost in human terms. Money isn't my primary concern. As you will see in the next chapter, my primary concern is to understand what I am doing and beyond that to care honestly about this person in front of me, who is not well. It's easy to recognize physicians who do this. You get the feeling that they have your best interests at heart.

Years ago I was working in a clinic for indigent people. It was a good match for them. The clinic looked indigent too. A psychiatrist with a strong regard for justice one day made the comment, "Look around. We embellish the things we value."

I do my best because that's a person sitting there in front of me, and a person has worth. How much money he has isn't the important thing. Besides, it's good practice to understand what you're doing and not make assumptions. It's just good medicine.

> I do my best because that's a person sitting there in front of me, and a person has worth. it's good practice to understand what you're doing and not make assumptions. It's just good medicine.

The movement from hostility to hospitality

Anger in the workplace is a hot topic today. When the doctor is something less than cordial, the chance of a happy ending is not good. Today we have therapists and coaches and all kinds of books and articles for what's called *anger management*.

If you ask me, anger is more than just a management problem. Just about anyone gets angry when victimized. Some people feel victimized by everything, so they're always angry. It's the way they see things. Then again, anger can have organic physical causes. Frontal brain tumors, traumatic brain injury and some forms of temporal lobe epilepsy can make a person suddenly break out in unprovoked rage. *Glass Half-empty* was born with dopamine chemistry in his brain that made him angry. The brain chemistry of manic illness does the same. Anger is just the final common pathway, a symptom, of a multitude of underlying causes, some biological, others psychological.

Beyond biology and psychology, the writings of Henri Nouwen[7] suggest that anger may be an expression of the spirit in which a person lives out his life. Nouwen's insight matches my own

> Anger may be an expression of the spirit in which a person lives out his life. Nouwen spoke of "a movement from hostility to hospitality" as a way of "creating a free and friendly space where the stranger can enter and become a friend instead of an enemy."

experience as well.

A compassionate and beloved priest, Nouwen spoke of "a movement from hostility to hospitality" as a way of "creating a free and friendly space where the stranger can enter and become a friend instead of an enemy." Although Nouwen saw this movement as "far from an easy task," I find that, though it may not be easy, there is a kind of simplicity about it.

The first part of this simplicity is awareness, becoming aware of the incredible power that our anger has over us. In the Grimm's fairytale we see how anger carries us along a path we don't want to take, as we cut off the heads of everyone we love, until we are sitting there, alone, saying over and over again, "What have I done!"

As I said a few paragraphs ago, admitting our anger and not making excuses for it puts it right out there in the open for all to see. By simply becoming aware, anger loses its power over us.

> Just say, "I'm sorry." In a cloaked way, it asks, "Please forgive me." More than cancer itself, carrying the guilt of never having been forgiven is a cancer that eats us up inside. It's an inborn part of every human being.

Once we have come to this painful awareness, and take back the power it had over us, we have a second simple task: to ask forgiveness. If that feels too religious for you, just say, "I'm sorry." Isn't that what saying you're sorry means anyway? It doesn't really mean that you're just sorry. In a cloaked way, it asks, "Please forgive me." More than cancer itself, carrying the guilt of never having been forgiven is a cancer that eats us up inside. I'm not talking religion here. This is archetypal. It's an inborn part of every human being.

These first two steps are simple and easy. The third step is simple, but not so easy. The *Glass Half-empty* fellow demonstrated it so well. It's gratitude. It's hard for anger to exist in the presence of gratitude. Gratitude is also one of the hardest things to feel when a person has been seriously victimized.

Anger, hostility, call it what you want. It's about gratitude and trust. How can I trust someone who wants to harm me? How could I not trust someone who I know cares about me? How can I provide care for someone as their doctor if the patient and I do not trust one another?

> Listening, looking into things and greeting the patient with a sense of hospitality is not management or religion or schmoozing, and it's more than just good doctoring. It's how a person says "I care about you." It's the beginning of trust.

There's a physician who refers to what I'm describing here as "schmoozing the patient." Nothing could be farther from the truth. Listening, looking into things and greeting the patient with a sense of hospitality is not management or religion or schmoozing, and it's more than just good doctoring. It's how a person says "I care about you." It's the beginning of trust, and that kind of trust is as vital to patient care with a good outcome as it is to the health of one's own family or any other relationship imaginable. It's built into our humanity. That's why it's so painful when it isn't there.

Curing and Healing

At first glance, the word curing suggests something we do with a pill or a surgical procedure, something like that. Healing means something different. It's the word that homeopathic medicine uses, a word that suggests herbals, vitamins, omega-3 and things like that.

Whether it's a pill or surgery or an herb, they're all cures to me, if they work that is. That's because they are all external things, things done to the patient from the outside. Here's an example of what I mean:

> *Foxtrot*: Imagine your headaches are cured, and now you are free to do all kinds of things that you would never attempt in your headache days. You say to yourself, "I'm ready to get with it and make some friends. I'm going to learn how to dance!"
>
> So you go to a studio and pay for foxtrot lessons. You happen to be the kind of person who says, "Just give me a pill, Doc. Then I'll be out of your hair." The doctor gave you a pill and your headaches went away. The doctor and his pill cured you.
>
> Now you're at the studio, and you go about learning the foxtrot in the same way. As you see it, learning to dance is something that the instructor does to you. The instructor pulls you up out of the chair. You're still bent at the waist, just like you were still sitting. So he pushes on your rear with one hand and on your shoulder with the other, so now you're standing straight. Then he adjusts you to dance posture, head over your spine.
>
> Next you have to step forward with your left foot, so he lifts your left foot and puts it where it needs to go, and so on and so forth.
>
> Just then someone comes in a few minutes late. This fellow wants to learn the foxtrot with a passion. "Sorry I'm late." He jumps right into position beside you, notices your posture, does the same and goes through all the steps, eagerly.

Who do you think will learn how to dance? Who's going to get nowhere and drop out after a lesson or two?

It doesn't matter whether you're learning the foxtrot, getting psychotherapy or getting rid of headaches. The person most likely to succeed is the person who participates, with a passion.

My mom and dad used a phrase that embodies this idea of participation. "David," they would say, "you have to learn how to stand on your own two feet and take care of yourself." Their job was to teach me how to do that. Their method was to give the locus of control to me. My parents were there to teach and to guide, but it was up to me to make the effort and the decisions.

They sent the message "I'll help you in any way I can." What does a child do with that? I fell in love with them and incorporated them. By the time I was 14, I was making decisions like my mom and dad. You didn't have to worry about me.

This "stand on your own two feet" idea was highly motivating because it put me in charge of myself at a young age. I wasn't passive and did not expect anyone to do my work. I understand that there are good psychological and biological reasons some individuals cannot do this. Even so, I urge you, as best you can, do not sit back and expect your doctor or therapist to do all the curing.

Don't expect to find wellness in a personal trainer, an herb, vitamin D or an organic tomato. Healing is something that happens within.

Healing in this way may not be an easy thing to do. Here's a better way to say it:

> With a disorder like migraine, the "cure" may not come in the form of a pill, but rather through a process of introspection and self-awareness. It can be as simple as taking on fewer projects at work or as complicated as mending an abusive relationship.
>
> One thing I would really hammer home is that this healing process can be a difficult task. Major life changes may be required. My concern is that the reader may come away not understanding the depth of the problem. In my days as a personal trainer, I remember an obese client who was clearly troubled by emotional issues. I made it clear that a person's mental state is as important to losing weight as exercise and diet. All he heard was the exercise and diet part. It's hard to confront the deep-seated issues that REALLY prevent true healing. Be sure your readers don't ignore that.
>
> Anonymous

I think he's trying to say that we don't find wellness in a personal trainer, an herb, vitamin D or an organic tomato. Healing is something that happens within.

———

It's odd. Relationships were so important in the success stories, yet we seldom talk about them.

Chapter Nine

To Answer the Question

A simple question has taken us on a long, unexpected journey, down a road less taken. Now where do we go?

I began by asking the pointed question: "Why do so many of us continue to live with headache?" By now you must be wondering, "So what's his answer?"

I learned some things about headache. Then the opening question took me on a long, unexpected journey. I set out to find what made a person better. Was it a medication? A special diet? Better sleep? Less stress? I was looking for the treatments that finally gave my patients a cure. What I found was far more important. In case after case the treatment was not the key to success. Asking "What made you better?" was the wrong question.

As if by chance, I stumbled upon a more important question: Why wasn't a correct diagnosis made in the first place? In other words, what kept you ill?

The answer to that was misdiagnosis most of the time. Simply stated, I found that headache was never the problem. Within the success stories, there was a single reason why so many of us continue to live with headaches. The treatments didn't work because they were treating the wrong thing. A flaw in the diagnosis of some kind was the culprit in nearly every case. When we finally understood the problem thoroughly, my patient got better.

Looking into why misdiagnosis occurred so often, I found that there was always an underlying cause that had been overlooked. That happened in many different ways. There were many obstacles to making a correct diagnosis.

Somehow, in the success stories when the patient finally became well, these obstacles were not there. I wanted to know just how the diagnosis was established with reasonable certainty in

> I set out asking, "What made you better?" That was the wrong question. What I found was far more important: "What kept you ill." A flaw in the diagnosis was the culprit in nearly every case.

> There were many obstacles to making a correct diagnosis. Somehow, when the patient finally became well, these obstacles were not there.

those cases. What was different about the process when we found the cure? The stories went on to show in detail how this happened.

Getting a correct diagnosis required a new way of thinking, one that focused on understanding the problem through and through. I even found a more sophisticated word for diagnosis: pathogenesis.

Getting a correct diagnosis required a new way of thinking and a good working relationship.

A second, less tangible, ingredient proved essential for success: a different kind of relationship between patient and doctor, one that embodied patient-centered care in the richest sense of the concept.

A good working relationship had a magical effect. In nearly every success story we had a mutual trust that allowed us to listen to one another to gain a better understanding of the illness. You might say there was a good spirit in the air.

We had a mutual trust that allowed us to listen to one another. You might say there was a good spirit in the air.

The relationship not only promoted a thorough understanding of the illness, it also fostered good judgement in its evaluation and treatment. This uncommon collaboration meant that *we* made the decisions, not the patient, not me and not the Academy of Neurology. The decisions were made by all of us together. No one was left out. There was a feeling of security, a feeling of safety in the relationship. The patient knew that I was committed to serving his or her best interests. When we could work together this way, that's when the magic happened. That's when the diagnosis was made, when the patient became well. At the heart of this good spirit was a movement away from depending on consensus guidelines toward looking to the patient for the answers.

If this is what it takes to get better, the question remains: "Can we do it?"

What It Takes

If it's going to take a new kind of thinking and a new style of working together, then how do we translate these ideas into action? It's like asking, "So, what's your business plan?"

One way to get a feel for what it takes might be to look at the office visit when we go down this road less taken. How does it differ? In my own experience, this different way of thinking and different kind of relationship is based on three essentials. They have to do with understanding what we are doing, using good judgement and something that I'd say is even more important, caring. Altogether, they make for a different kind of office visit.

Understanding what we are doing, good judgement and caring, altogether, they make for a different kind of office visit.

Understanding

One theme came across loud and clear in nearly every success story. The headaches eluded a cure because they were misdiagnosed. Although we saw this happen in many ways, they all add up to a single directive: we need to understand what we are doing. Understanding what we are doing, exactly what does that mean?

By now, you can see that it isn't so simple, this matter of understanding. It's easier to just treat symptoms without the understanding part. The movement toward understanding has two essential ingredients: first, a simple change in focus and second, learning new diagnostic skills. The second part is not so simple.

Focus on root cause: Rather than move straight into treating the headache, we need to think of the headache as only a symptom, and turn our attention to finding the root cause of the symptom. Our approach changes dramatically because our efforts turn from treating to diagnosing. We stay focused on finding the diagnosis until we know the cause of the headache. This change in focus alone makes the office visit look quite different.

> Rather than move straight into treating the headache, we need to think of the headache as only a symptom, and turn our attention to finding the root cause of the symptom.

As the patient is saying, "All I want is a pill." and goes on to tell me what other physicians have done, I find myself saying, "But they're all treatments. I don't want to talk about treatment because we don't even know what we'd be treating. Let's get back to finding the cause. So tell me more about . . ."

If we were to focus on treating symptoms, I would have prescribed medications and discussed non-medication therapies. I might have counseled the patient. On the other hand, if we focus on finding the underlying cause, we use the visit to look into things. We get more history, do medication trials, order diagnostic studies and so forth. When there's concern about a tumor, we naturally go into diagnosis-mode. It's just as important to search for the underlying cause when we're evaluating one of the benign headaches, especially when it's migraine.

When a person says, "Doc, I've tried so many things. I just want to know what's causing these headaches." I'm thinking, "Right on!" Here's someone who understands the need to focus on diagnosis and stay there until we understand what's going on.

Diagnostic skills: Diagnosing requires some skills. Without them, it would have been nearly impossible to bring many of the cases presented here to a happy ending.

When everyone is asking "How are we going to fix this?" The engineer in me is wondering "How are we going to figure this out?" If that's the focus, then you spend your day trying to find new ways to figure things out. If you're diagnosis-minded, you'll find many, many ways to figure things out. With time, your repertoire of diagnostic tricks gets bigger and bigger and your skill in using them grows accordingly. This is what diagnosticians and engineers do best.

> **When everyone is asking "How are we going to fix this?" The engineer in me is wondering "How are we going to figure this out?"**

You've seen in the headache stories how some of these diagnostic techniques are used. For example, diagnostic medication trials were essential to establishing the diagnosis in the cases of basilar artery migraine, migraine activated by the manic disorder and even in migraine activated by worry. In the case of *Special Ed* an anticonvulsant was diagnostic. In *Glass Half-empty* the failure of so many medication trials told me what he didn't have. Finally the Haldol trial proved what the cause really was: something I had never seen before. A single dose of Ambien in *One of My Pills* showed exactly why this woman couldn't get rid of her headaches. In other cases we learned how to apply other diagnostic methods. The Wright Brothers principle and the correlation technique helped establish the pathogenesis in several cases.

When the symptoms went away for *Seven Years of Hell*, I suggested she stop the verapamil to see if it was really what made her better. She wanted no part of that. So I said, "Well then, stay on it for a year or two. If you're completely free of symptoms for that long a time, and the symptoms come back when you miss some doses, then you'll have convincing evidence that indeed your symptoms were caused by vasospasm. You'll learn something no matter what you do."

In the same way, recognizing psychosocial forces driving headache is a valuable diagnostic skill that's necessary to understand what we are doing. Regarding psychosocial skills: The word I would use is indispensable. We can't do without them.

The lack of diagnostic skills is like being an airline pilot, and you're not too good at flying. I think poor diagnostic skills, especially the psychosocial ones, is often behind the patient who is dismissed as "You need to see a psychiatrist." It's easy to give the patient a psychiatric diagnosis, by default, when you can't figure out the problem.

At the other extreme, failure to recognize the emotional part of an illness accounts for an enormous amount of misdiagnosis and suffering. Just look at *Vivacious* who went 20 years with untreatable migraine because the manic trait was below the threshold of detection for all the doctors who had gone before. An indispensable psychosocial skill is the ability to put yourself in someone else's shoes, and honor the fact that that's a person there in front of you. Should we call that caring? The two are hard to separate.

But please keep one thought in mind. Not everyone is cut out for diagnostic medicine. It's a talent. Some have a knack for it, some don't. Just as you wouldn't want me doing surgery on you, in the same sense, everyone doesn't need to be a diagnostician. Some are better in other roles. Nevertheless, *somebody* needs to know how to fly the plane. We simply must see the value of diagnosis.

> **Not everyone is cut out for diagnostic medicine. It's a talent. Everyone doesn't need to be a diagnostician. We simply must see the value of diagnosis.**

Good judgement

A second, less obvious, theme in the stories had to do with judgement. It goes without saying that anyone who cares for patients must use their best judgement, always.

> *Against My Better Judgement:* Some years ago I heard of a physician who was in court defending himself in a malpractice lawsuit. He was on the witness stand and had taken the oath to tell "the truth, the whole truth, and nothing but the truth," when the plaintiff's lawyer asked, "Doctor so and so, tell me, what was your thinking when you prescribed that medication for your patient?"
>
> Intimidated by the question, and without a thought, he quickly answered, "Well, to be honest, I didn't want to prescribe the medication. It was against my better judgement. But the patient was so insistent . . ."
>
> The attorney's next question: "Why would you *ever* do anything against your better judgement?"

It sounds simple enough, always using your better judgement, doesn't it? Believe me it isn't. That's because different people have different judgements. What *I* consider good judgement may not be what *you* call good judgement. So who decides?

Do no harm: There is an honored tradition on graduating from medical school. Just before the doctorate is given, the medical school class recites the Hippocratic Oath, a code of conduct in the practice of medicine to which the new physician pledges obedience. If there is anything we remember from the oath, it's the promise to "do no harm." In the practice of medicine, it's the Golden Rule, the ultimate standard upon which we base medical ethics.

"Do no harm." is no empty promise. It's the first consideration in weighing the risk versus benefit of any diagnostic procedure or treatment. It's a principle we use every day, but it isn't always clear just what it's telling us to do. Here's how it works.

> *Ominous:* Imagine a 16 year-old girl who presents with an ominous form of multiple sclerosis.[10] She's losing bladder control and is barely able to walk, so she probably has had a spinal cord attack. She had seen a neurologist who ordered some scans, made the diagnosis and recommended a safe but low efficacy medicine to slow the progression.
>
> The patient and her family came for a second opinion. They wanted to know, "What's the best thing to do?"
>
> Do we use a treatment that approaches 100% efficacy and is tolerated well, but carries a risk of a life-threatening brain infection or do we use a safe treatment only 30% effective and not likely to arrest progression in a case like this? To one person do no harm tells us to use the low efficacy treatment. Even though she winds up in a wheelchair, smelling like urine by the time she's 30, at least your treatment hasn't harmed her. Another person might say that, in fact, you *did* harm the patient because you knew her chances with the MS weren't good, and you probably could have arrested the MS with the high-efficacy medication.
>
> I can't just say, "You decide. It's up to you." They're worried. They don't know what to do. "Dr. Smith, is there anything that might help? Do you have any ideas?"

They've told me the story, I've done an exam and now the patient and her parents want to hear what I have to say. It comes down to "Should we use the safe treatment? Is the more effective treatment worth the risk? What should we do?"

To continue the story, our first encounter might go something like this.

> I'm thinking, "I need to see for myself how bad this

"Do no harm." is no empty promise. It's the first consideration in weighing the risk versus benefit of any diagnostic procedure or treatment.

10. **Multiple sclerosis (MS)** is a neurological disorder in which a person's immune system repeatedly attacks the brain, spinal cord and optic nerves. Without treatment, it often progresses to disability. Today we have quite effective ways to prevent this from happening.

is." So I ask, "Could you get a copy of the scans and come back tomorrow? I want to look at them."

The next day they're back in my office. I have the MRI scans up on the screen and Mom comments, "Oh this is interesting. We haven't seen these." I'm wondering if the neurologist who ordered the scans even took a look at them.

It's a low resolution study of the head and cervical spine and done with a technique that would be a poor measure of MS at best. The brain shows large, active areas of demyelination. It's MS all right. It looks like there might be an MS plaque at the top of the spinal cord, but I can't be sure. The images were so poor that you couldn't see a spinal cord plaque if it was there.

The situation is ominous. An aggressive pattern like this at 16 does not have a good outlook. Unless we arrest the MS, she will likely be in a wheelchair by the time she's 30.

"These don't have enough detail to make a treatment decision; how about another scan?"

I ordered a high resolution MRI using a protocol that the radiologist and I have optimized for MS. The spinal cord images are as good as they get. Now we clearly see a big MS plaque at the top of the spinal cord and several others elsewhere in the cord. The situation is ominous. An aggressive pattern like this at 16 does not have a good outlook. Unless we arrest the MS, she will likely be in a wheelchair by the time she's 30. There's no going back from there.

Turning to my patient and her family, "Tell me what you're thinking. How do you feel about what you see here?"

I influenced the decision to be sure, but I did not make the decision. It was a decision that *we* made.

The conversation goes on from there. They have questions. I answer them the best I can, making it clear that there are uncertainties. Talking back and forth like this, we come to a decision. It's like the "None of us is as smart as all of us." principle that Craig, my brother-in-law, uses. We do a great deal of listening, both ways. I influenced the decision to be sure, but I did not make the decision. It was a decision that *we* made.

Do no harm just doesn't seem enough here; there needs to be a better way of saying that medical care is, or is not, good care.

Who's to say?

Take a minute to look back over this story. Would you say that the first neurologist did a good job? He did no harm; or did he? Do no harm just doesn't seem enough here; there needs to be a better way of saying that medical care is, or is not, good care.

What constitutes good care anyway? The answer depends on who you ask.

Others say: More often than I care to admit, I've heard it said, "Smith, he does too much testing and those medications he prescribes are too expensive." One physician in town took it a little further, "Smith, he's driving our healthcare system into bankruptcy." I'm sure he would quickly point out the cost of her second set of MRI scans and the very high cost of the MS treatment.

I think it's safe to call this the prevailing opinion today, at least among those responsible for managing and paying for our medical care. It's expensive business, giving care, if we want to do it well.

I say: As I see it, the consequences of not fixing the problem the first time are far more costly than anything I suggest here. It's like putting a roof on a house. If you don't do it right at the outset, it's going to cost more in the long run. In the long run, doing it right the first time is a bargain in terms of both dollars and cents and human misery.

Oddly, it isn't often that I hear someone complain about the quality of an MRI. Maybe that's because those who order the studies don't look at what they get. True, a scan can be of poor quality for a number of unavoidable reasons. *Ominous*, however, had a poor quality scan one day, then ten days later had a scan of superb quality. This is not rare in my experience. As you saw in this case, the consequences can be serious. We're not talking about a roof here; we're talking about a person.

My contribution in this case was to make an effort to get the first MRI scans and take the time to look at the images with the patient and her family. The study was not of sufficient quality to make a treatment decision. What's more, the patient and her family were not even aware of that fact or its importance to her future. To make a well-founded decision, we had to know how serious this was. High resolution MRI revealed an ominous situation. She was clearly in trouble. Knowing that, we could weigh the risks of the MS against the risks and benefits of treatment. Then we could make a good treatment decision.

Ordering a scan without the best technique in a case like this is not good medicine. It isn't just bad care, it's unacceptable. It's a recipe for disability, disability that does not have to happen, and

> **What constitutes good care anyway? The answer depends on who you ask.**

it's a waste of money. I wondered, "Did he look at the scans? Did he even care?"

We all make mistakes. It's especially not good to make a mistake if you're a doctor or an airline pilot, but they happen even when you try your best. You might call these "errors made in good faith." Then there is harm that comes by malicious intent and there is harm caused by negligence. None are good; but where do we place the harm that occurs simply because we don't care? It isn't negligent or malicious, and not caring is not what you'd call "good faith." In my judgement, harm that comes from not caring is somewhere between malicious harm and negligence. Not caring is another thing we don't want in a doctor or an airline pilot for that matter.

Why did I make an effort to understand what's going on? That's easy. One simple sentence says it all. "I care about you." Caring goes beyond saying, "My first duty is to the patient in my charge." because caring isn't a duty. It's something higher than that. If I care about a person, naturally, I want to do my best for him.

An interesting thing happens when I make an effort to understand the problem thoroughly at the outset. A correct diagnosis leads to good treatment decisions from the beginning. Usually the patient does well, and then he or she really *doesn't need me* any more.

When I make an effort to understand the problem thoroughly at the outset, a correct diagnosis leads to good treatment decisions, the patient does well and then he or she really doesn't need me anymore.

Patients say: In 35 years of practice I haven't heard many patients regret a thorough workup. Most feel that it's in their best interests. What do they have to say? Listen on to some if the things I've heard patients say.

> *Scant Visit:* A man in his 40s saw a physician for bad headaches. He's worried. "They started a week ago. I never get headaches."
>
> The response from his physician: "Oh it's probably just your allergies. Here, take this." He writes a script for an allergy medication. "Come back if it doesn't help."
>
> A new headache is a red flag for a potentially serious underlying cause: aneurysm, sleep apnea and so on. We saw him a few days later and ordered bloodwork to rule out a medical problem, an MRI to rule out a brain tumor and overnight pulse oximetry to rule out obstructive sleep apnea. All came back normal except the pulse ox, which showed severe sleep apnea. CPAP fixed that, and the

headaches went away.

The first physician saw the patient without a wait. The visit ended on time, and it generated a note that justified the bill, but the patient would have been just as well off if the visit had never happened. The physician responsible for the person's welfare made no attempt to find the cause. He pulled an answer out of thin air for a headache that clearly requires investigation. After a visit like this, one patient commented, "Nothing of substance was accomplished."

Another patient put it this way: "I've seen six doctors for this problem. You're the first one who brings his brain to the office every morning." Saying it more kindly, another commented, "The mystery is still better than a wrong diagnosis." By the way, it was an engineer who said that.

One of my patients expressed the futility of this kind of care when she left her doctor muttering "I have horrible headaches. You don't know what I've got. And you tell me to try this pill and come back in three months!" Another patient calls them "make-believe doctors!" That's quite an allegation for a profession whose responsibility is the welfare of persons. I think they were trying to say that the doctors were not serving their best interests.

It's easy to see how doing less makes sense from a management or business point of view, but it doesn't work at all in the medicine-as-a-caring-profession kind of model.

It's easy to see how doing less makes sense from a management or business point of view. The visit is simpler. The patient gets in and out on time. You don't spend much money on tests and, the less you do, the less chance there is of doing harm.

Doing less fits the medicine-as-a-business model quite well, but it doesn't work at all in the medicine-as-a-caring-profession kind of model. In the practice of medicine, a simple error of omission can do great harm.

From following to understanding: Here we see three definitions of good judgement: 1) follow the consensus of experts, 2) understand through and through and 3) just give me some help. Who's right? Most physicians would agree that the best thing to do is to follow guidelines because they are based on the best evidence we have.

"What Should We Be Doing?" Imitrex was introduced in 1993. Soon after, I saw a man for chronic dizziness who made it very clear that the problem was dizziness. "I don't have headaches." He wasn't able to describe the dizziness

very well. It was a vague kind of thing. No cause was found by a thorough evaluation in a dizziness lab.

He was sensitive to light, felt "Blah." and just looked ill in general. Medical evaluation and scans were normal. I said that I had seen migraine do this before. I offered an Imitrex injection. He accepted.

The next morning he called. "What was in that miracle shot? I haven't felt this good in ages!" I later found the cause of the migraine and treated that.

A few days after the Imitrex shot his PCP called, appreciative. "So what should we be doing now, Dave, using Imitrex as first line therapy?" Our guideline at that time was to use Imitrex only when all else fails.[11]

I thought, "I don't know what we should be doing. Maybe we should be thinking about our patients, trying to understand what's going on."

Incidentally, the Imitrex guideline is long gone.

Why do we have guidelines? I see two good reasons. First, there's the matter of safety. Guidelines help to protect the patient. Without guidelines, how do I know what's best? That's a physician's ever-present concern in caring for a person. Whether I'm discussing the plan at the end of a visit or talking to someone on the phone, every day I find myself asking, "What's the best thing to do in this situation?" Guidelines not only say that it's acceptable to apply a recipe to our cases, they suggest that the recipe is usually the best thing to do.

This brings us to a second reason for guidelines. They clearly spell out what we *should* do during a visit, and clearly define the evaluation and treatment. We don't have to do so much thinking, and we can rest secure. If anything goes wrong, we can always say, "Well, I gave the standard of care."

That isn't what we did in the **Ominous** case. When it came to using "my better judgement," my guideline was simple: It's always best to make an effort to understand the illness. Especially when the diagnosis is uncertain or when the illness is ominous, it's unnerving to apply someone else's recipe. I'm thinking, "I better find out what's going on here."

When I don't know what's going on, I stay in diagnostic-mode and continue to search for an answer to the mystery. Following someone else's guideline tends to push inquiry aside. It excludes

We need a better way to judge how well we are serving our patients' best interests.

11. Step therapy, also known as *step edit*, is an attempt to control medication costs and risks by using the least expensive, safest medications first, then progressing to more costly, higher risk medications if they don't work. There's debate as to how effective this is. The story here shows how, in just one visit, the use of an expensive brand medication as first line diagnosis-treatment brought an end to a long line of expensive evaluations and failed treatments.

the process of discovery. As we saw with Lamictal in the case of *Vivacious*, if we just follow and don't think for ourselves, the guidelines actually may prevent us from doing the best thing.

When we change from thinking that the problem is the headache to it's never the headache, we've already departed from today's practice guidelines. They tell us to treat the migraine and even what medications to use. The longer we stay in diagnostic-mode, the farther we depart from guidelines. The first change in our thinking, diagnosis first, has forced a second change, the change from following to understanding.

When we change from thinking that the problem is the headache to it's never the headache, we've already departed from today's practice guidelines.

Anything goes: "Wow!" you're thinking. "If it's all up to my best judgement, then anything goes. No rules. No consequences. I like this guy. I can just say that it was a judgement call." A more acceptable way to say "Anything goes!" might be to say "It's all relative. My judgement is not your judgement." True, there's an element of uncertainty in nearly every medical decision, but that doesn't mean that one decision is as good as another. Some outcomes are better than others.

The first change in our thinking, diagnosis first, has forced a second change, the change from following to understanding.

Judgement Call: What if things go sour after the *Scant Visit*, and harm comes to the patient in some way? Suppose someone says, "An MRI is clearly indicated for a new and unusual headache like this." You can always say, "Well, he had a stuffy nose. In my best judgement, it was allergy. I made a judgement call."

A judgement call, what's that? One of the best definitions I've come across defines it this way:

> "If you refer to a decision as a judgement call, you mean that there are no firm rules or principles that can help you make it, so you simply have to rely on your own judgement and instinct"[12]

The definition says that one makes a judgement call when there are no firm rules. That's odd. The patient didn't think it was good judgement, even as he walked out of the office, and that was before any consequence. Did he know something the doctor didn't know? Was he using some principle not in the guideline?

Yes, if you asked the patient to explain why he was upset after the scant visit, he might say, "I was hoping that the doctor would have more interest in my welfare. I was hoping he'd care."

12. **Judgment call;** http:\\ dictionary.reverso.net/ english-cobuild/judgment call. Accessed 11/14/2013.

Caring

Becoming well, whether you're the one with the headaches or the one who's trying to help, goes beyond just knowing this and that. Doing some good in this world requires something more than understanding and good judgement. A third theme emerged from the success stories that, I'm sure, is obvious to most, but seldom mentioned in any discussion of migraine : a good spirit between patient and doctor. In Chapter Eight I called this a style of working together.

> **Grand Fellow:** Returning to the author of the *Only 20 Minutes* story, Dr. Joynt had more than mere wisdom.
>
> I remember hearing Dr. Joynt deliver a eulogy for Norman Geshwind, his colleague and friend who had been a great teacher and had made substantial contributions to the field of neurology. Joynt said that there was an old celtic way to describe a person like Geshwind: "He was a grand fellow." Dr. Joynt was trying to say that Geshwind had something more than wisdom. He had a kind heart.

When he said that, I thought, "You're talking about yourself, Dr. Joynt." As a teacher, department chair, as a physician and as a person, Joynt had something beyond wisdom. He had a selfless regard for all those about him. At the root of it, he was a caring man, a grand fellow indeed.

Dr. Joynt left behind a lesson for us all. By listening to a patient, a colleague, or anyone for that matter, by having concern for a person's best interests, by doing our best, we honor the worth of the person. They are universal signs of caring. If we want to help someone, how far can we go without caring?

A rich learning environment: Even in three years of training, I didn't find it easy to acquire all the knowledge and skills and judgement one needs to practice good neurology. There's a lot to learn. While it may not be easy, it is indeed possible for a training program to turn out highly competent physicians.

But what about caring? How do we learn that? Watching pre-med students begin their journey, I can see that it will take more than a course in ethics, a medical school rotation through psychiatry or some kind of program. Caring is a kind of maturation that has as much to do with the learning environment as it does

Doing some good in this world requires something more than understanding and good judgement.

By listening, by having concern for a person's best interests, by doing our best, we honor the worth of the person. They are universal signs of caring. If we want to help someone, how far can we go without caring?

the person embedded that environment trying to learn something. It's a process, a quest.

MIT: At MIT I found myself in one of the richest learning environments imaginable. There, our professors referred to us beginners as "the cream of the crop." I felt valued. In another school one could get by with memorizing and cramming for exams. At MIT memorizing didn't work. Understanding wasn't just required, it was revered.

Caring is a maturation, a process, a quest.

After leaving MIT and returning to the real world, I remember how disillusioned I felt. I asked myself, "What's missing out here?" Then after medical school, I had two learning experiences that brought back the good feeling, experiences pivotal in forming my approach to the patient. I began to understand what it was that the real world was missing.

Eye Clinic: In 1977, as I was finishing neurology residency, Dr. Joynt offered me a position in the Department of Neurology. A few days later, I had my glasses checked in the Ophthalmology Department. The department had just moved into the entire first floor of the new outpatient wing and had some rooms to spare. The resident checking my eyes raised her brow and said, "Why not put your office here? It would be great to have a neurologist around." One thing led to another. Before I knew it, I had become the Neuro-ophthalmology Service at the University hospital. That led to the first of these two remarkable learning experiences.

In the Eye Clinic, for my first 12 years of practice, I offered curbside neurology consults to the residents and ophthalmologists, but what they gave me in return was far more. To be sure, I saw many common and strange ophthalmology cases, and I learned quite a bit. However, it was *how* the learning occurred that was so remarkable.

The Eye Clinic was a collegial kind of place. We were all friends there, and we had a great deal of respect for one another. Don Zehl, the retina specialist, might knock on my door with a neuro question. I'd always say, "Where's the patient now?"

"She's in my office." We'd walk 20 feet to his exam room, and see the patient together. I always come away having learned more about retina than I could ever have taught him about neurology. Again, I felt valued. So the learning was about more than just being taught something. It was mentoring of the very best kind. One year of that was all I needed to know that neuro-ophthalmology was my destiny.

Biopsychosocial Fellowship: A few years after I left the University for private practice, I had another fortunate opportunity, the second learning experience. This time it took the form of a post-doctoral fellowship in the biopsychosocial (BPS) approach to the patient.

George Engel had started the idea 50 years earlier. He was an internist who had set up practice in the psychiatry department. He authored *The Clinical Approach to the Patient*, the bible to every third year medical student when we saw patients for the first time.

I spent two years embedded in an environment with physicians and a clinical psychologist who had incredible insight into patients and the physicians who care for them. Again, I was highly valued.

Engel taught that a person's illness was more than a biological problem. There were always psychological and social components to an illness that needed to be understood and factored into the treatment. He established the hospital's Med-Psych Liaison Service based on this idea. Engel's biopsychosocial fellows, internists he trained in his approach, provided the consultations. Incidentally, when we neurology residents needed an in-patient psych consult, we didn't call psychiatry. We called the med-psych liaison. They gave better consults.

When I took the fellowship myself, it was largely run by Engel's former fellows, but Engel was still teaching, and I had an opportunity to discuss cases with him. It was like becoming a third year medical student all over again, after 15 years of practice, but this time I was doing it right. I spent two years embedded in an environment with physicians and a clinical psychologist who had incredible insight into patients and the physicians who care for them. Again, I was highly valued.

The Magic: There was some kind of magic happening in the Eye Clinic and in the BPS fellowship. My mentors and the environment they created promoted the best kind of learning. There was no competition, no intimidation with one-upmanship and no defensiveness. No one ever spoke over me, ever. It was easy to say, "I don't know that." and go on to learn what I didn't know. I could pursue my interests in the healthiest way imaginable. These learning environments held me in high esteem and harkened back to MIT where the professors called us "the cream of the crop."

Sometimes I wonder how many physicians have the good fortune to train in this way. I think I know the answer. It shows in the stories my patients tell. When they say how many doctors they've seen over years for headaches that fell apart quickly when I spotted the psychosocial activators or began to use medication trials for diagnosis. It tells me that somehow their physicians missed out on something important.

Nevertheless, I'm certain that what they may have missed are *teachable* skills. I'm sure of this because even my pre-med clinical assistants begin to show good psychosocial skills after they've been embedded in the clinic environment here for a few months. Please don't think that clinical assistants make the diagnoses here. I'm the one who does that. I'm trying to say that, in fact, it is possible to acquire impressive clinical skills and to do so rapidly. Caring takes longer, but there is an environment that promotes the trait.

Just what is this magic that allows an emerging physician to acquire the skills he needs so rapidly? Is it something tangible? Is there a principle? An attitude? Is there something we can do to make a good learning environment happen at will?

I believe that Henri Nouwen hit the nail on the head when he spoke of the movement from hostility to hospitality. He was saying that it is *we* who create the free and friendly space where a stranger can enter and become a friend. It's as easy and as hard as that. *We* are the magic.

At MIT, I developed an innate need to figure things out so that I could understand. You might even say that it was there that the trait began to mature; it became a reverence for understanding. In the Eye Clinic I learned quite a bit about ophthalmology and medicine in general, but those 12 years gave me something even more important. I watched as my mentors expressed caring. I witnessed Nouwen's idea of a free and friendly space applied to the practice of medicine. After the BPS fellowship, I could recognize and understand much better the psychosocial factors in a person's illness. Beyond that, I think it helped me personally. It allowed me to give something better to my patients.

A good learning environment is about more than just learning science. What happens when someone says that you're the cream

> There was some kind of magic happening in the Eye Clinic and in the BPS fellowship. These learning environments held me in high esteem and harkened back to MIT where the professors called us "the cream of the crop."

of the crop or becomes your friend and mentor and makes you feel highly valued? When a mentor treats the student with such high regard, he is showing him how to have regard for another person. By example, the student is learning how to bring hospitality into the practice of medicine.

I'm certain that caring is teachable and I know well the environment in which that occurs, but experience tells me, "doing what it takes" to foster caring will be quite some challenge.

A New Culture

My attempt to understand why so many are plagued with headache has brought us well beyond this thin slice of medical care. A simple question about headache has taken us on a long, unexpected journey that brings us face-to-face with how medical care is given today. We've had a glimpse, even some insight, into medical care in general.

I learned something about what cures headaches, then realized that the cure wasn't what I needed to know; it was finding the underlying cause. That's what made a person well.

Along the way I stumbled on something of paramount importance: I began to see exactly how misdiagnosis happens. While searching each case for the pathogenesis of headache, I found the pathogenesis of medical error as well. It was clear that we need some changes.

Guiding principles

If you agree that we need some changes, then what should they be? What principles should guide the way? The stories here speak, in a compelling way, to what patients want and don't want in medical care. There's no uncertain direction here. They give us a guiding principle that must be the foundation for any change, any decision, and any judgement that we make. To make things right, we will need to go beyond "Do no harm."

In its most elementary form, my patients and their stories are begging for a guiding principle that emphasizes three fundamentals of patient care.

> In providing medical care, we must understand the patient's illness to the best of our ability, use our best judgement and, above all, we must care about the person

---

When a mentor treats the student with high regard, he is showing him how to have regard for another person. By example, the student is learning how to bring hospitality into the practice of medicine.

While searching for the pathogenesis of headache, I found the pathogenesis of medical error as well.

It was clear that we need to go beyond "Do no harm."

whose welfare is in our hands.

Thomas Jefferson might have called these "self-evident truths." I think of them as *timeless* truths. They are fundamentals that follow naturally from the idea of patient-centered care.

This precept contains the imperative to "do no harm," but makes it much more clear what that really means. It tells me not only what I should *not* do, but also what I *should* do.

A theory in need of proof

In Chapter One I promised a fresh look at headaches, from the perspective of an engineer. I think I've done that. I said that it's time for a change, and wound up with a simple directive for good medical care, a directive based on understanding, good judgement and caring.

We must understand the patient's illness to the best of our ability, use our best judgement and, above all, we must care about the person whose welfare is in our hands.

It's easy to say, "We need more of this or more of that." However, it isn't necessarily easy to provide everything we need. Resources have limits and there are many in need. That's simply a reality that has to be factored into any plan we make for better care. It's a matter of allocating resources.

Few would disagree with allocating resources to serve the greater good, but when we try to do that, that's when the heated debate comes. There's debate because no one knows with certainty what constitutes good care. Then sentiment and opinion and special interests take control. Endless debate stymies any real progress, and it's costly. If we knew for sure what was best, the debate would end, for the most part, and we could move forward to do our best in every sense of the word.

No one knows with certainty what constitutes good care. If we knew for sure what was best, we could move forward to do our best in every sense of the word.

There is an interesting precedent for a situation like this.

> *T Zone:* I remember, as a first year medical student, looking through the archives of the Journal of the American Medical Society in the basement of the medical library. I don't remember what I was looking for, but I'll never forget my surprise to see an ad for Camel cigarettes right there in a medical journal. The ad showed a confident physician with cigarette in hand. In large print it read "According to a recent Nationwide survey: More Doctors smoke Camels than any other cigarette." At the bottom of the ad was a picture of a woman, also with a cigarette in hand. A T-shaped box drawn over her upper airway had the words "You're T-Zone will tell you . . ." as it

11. Oppenheimer GM. Becoming the Framingham Study 1947-1950. *Am J Public Health,* 2005 April; 95(4): 602-610.

went on to say how mild Camels are for your throat.

That issue of JAMA was published in the early 1950s. By 1953 JAMA and the New England Journal of Medicine had banned all tobacco ads. Why the change? It had to do with proof.

As antibiotics became available in the 1940s, infection as a cause of death dropped dramatically. Death due to cardiovascular disease (heart attack) then became a primary concern. The problem was that no one knew what to do about it. There was no solid understanding of its cause.

Hoping to get some answers, the Framingham Study was begun in 1948.[11] A cohort of residents in this small Massachusetts town was selected to be studied over a period of years. to better understand the cause(s) of cardiovascular disease. Within a few years they had mounting evidence that smoking tobacco contributed strongly to the development of cardiovascular disease. As I said, the major medical journals banned cigarette ads in 1953. In the 1960s we saw a decline in death from cardiovascular disease, largely due to insight from the Framingham study.

> **From the Framingham study we had a clear direction with a measurable impact.**

Finally we knew something with enough confidence to take the steam out of the debate. From the Framingham study we had a clear direction for prevention that had a measurable impact on mortality from cardiovascular disease.

New Framingham

I've made quite a few assertions here, and I realize they need proving. Clearly, there needs to be a study. It needs to be a *good* study, one that doesn't make assumptions and is not easily manipulated by special interests. It needs to have enough credibility to end the debate and give a clear direction.

Imagine a community-based study done over a period of years. In this way it would be similar to the Framingham study. However, instead of trying to understand cardiovascular disease, this new study would bring some understanding to medical care, how it's provided, that is. One way to do this might be to introduce into a community a group of physicians dedicated to the principles of patient-centered care proposed here. Then make a side-by-side comparison of this group with the community's existing health care system(s).

> **There needs to be a *good* study, one with enough credibility to end the debate and give a clear direction.**

To be of any value, this "New Framingham" study would have to incorporate the ideas described in The Best of Both Worlds

(Chapter Seven). It would have to combine non-parametric and parametric methods in such a way that non-parametric methods discover the important questions and parametric methods answer these questions with a high degree of confidence.

For example, we might ask, "Is it true that misdiagnosis is as common and as costly as Smith believes?" That's a question raised by the non-parametric methods used here. It would be interesting to measure the cost of care when a person's headaches were misdiagnosed and compare this to the cost of the evaluation that established a definitive diagnosis. That should say something about the performance of a medical care system and its providers.

We might measure the migration rate of patients from one system to the another. Here we'd have an interesting measure of patient satisfaction. The possibilities are endless. This might be a reliable way to test the impact of new ideas in medical care and new technologies as they emerge.

Less traveled

You may be thinking "Well, hasn't this been done?" Mayo and Cleveland Clinics, among others, are committed to thorough diagnostic evaluation and patient-centered care. Furthermore, they already have practice groups in outlying communities.

I agree, in part. True, a number of medical centers use the approach I suggest here. In fact, I send patients to them when I can't make a diagnosis. Nevertheless, debate continues. The question remains, "Are the extensive evaluations of Mayo and Cleveland running us into bankruptcy or not?" Some say "Yes!" adamantly. Other say "Absolutely not! It's the best care and it's cost-effective."

As long as we hear such intense difference of opinion, we know that we are trying to make healthcare decisions based on opinion, not fact.

As long as we hear such intense difference of opinion, we know that we are trying to make healthcare decisions based on opinion, not fact. The debate will never end until we have undeniable evidence that one way is better than another. We'll be stymied and without direction until the important questions are answered with a high degree of certainty. Incontrovertible evidence will end the debate. New Framingham would provide that.

Let me say again, a New Framingham study must begin with a non-parametric method to open the door to the important questions. Only then would quantitative, parametric studies give answers that we can trust. So a study like this must be led by individuals skilled in patient-centered care. Paradoxically, our patients' stories, mere anecdote, would become the source of the most important evidence.

Placing different care paradigms side-by-side, comparing them this way, intuitively seems to be a realistic and powerful way to understand good medical care. If one is clearly superior, it should be obvious. How could it not grow and become a new culture of medical care?

A New Framingham study will require a break with tradition, if it is to test new ideas. Different thinking and a different style add up to taking a different path, don't they? The road, which today is less taken, may tomorrow bring us to a new culture in medical care. If it leads to better care, and if it's affordable, I can only expect that it would grow to become the new standard of care. Oddly, the road less traveled might become the road that someday everyone wants to take.

> **The road, which today is less taken, may tomorrow become the road that someday everyone wants to take.**

Coming to the end of *The Road Not Taken*, Frost closed with the words:

> Two roads diverged in a wood, and I -
> I took the one less traveled by,
> And that has made all the difference.

I know how he must have felt. I can only say the same.